OSTEOLOGY FOR RADIOGRAPHERS

This book is dedicated to
the memory of my Dad

OSTEOLOGY FOR RADIOGRAPHERS

Christina Shillingford
TDCR, DipEd
Deputy Principal
Schools of Radiography and Radiotherapy
Guy's Hospital, London

Blackwell Scientific Publications
OXFORD LONDON EDINBURGH
BOSTON PALO ALTO MELBOURNE

Editorial Offices:
Osney Mead, Oxford, OX2 0EL
8 John Street, London, WC1N 2ES
23 Ainslie Place, Edinburgh, EH3 6AJ
52 Beacon Street, Boston, Massachusetts 02108, USA
667 Lytton Avenue, Palo Alto, California 94301, USA
107 Barry Street, Carlton, Victoria 3053, Australia

First published 1985

Set by Burns & Smith, Derby
Printed and bound by Billing and Sons Ltd, Worcester

DISTRIBUTORS

USA
Blackwell Mosby Book Distributors
11830 Westline Industrial Drive
St Louis, Missouri 63141

Canada
Blackwell Mosby Book Distributors
120 Melford Drive, Scarborough
Ontario M1B 2X4

Australia
Blackwell Scientific Publications (Australia) Pty Ltd
107 Barry Street, Carlton
Victoria 3053

British Library
Cataloguing in Publication Data

Shillingford, Christina
Osteology for radiographers.
1. Skeleton—Radiography
I. Title
611'.71'024616 QM101

ISBN 0-632-01349-4

CONTENTS

PREFACE

This book was written primarily for students studying for the Diploma of the College of Radiographers' (DCR) examination. Osteology is an important section of the syllabus and, at present, there is a dearth of concise quick-reference texts at the required level of knowledge for the student of radiography to consult.

My aim is to guide the students through their study of the bones of the skeleton by including relevant information only, simplifying the diagrams as much as possible and linking anatomy with pathology. The approach to the study of individual bones follows a logical sequence throughout the book, thereby encouraging the student to do likewise. Self-tests are included to encourage students to assess their acquired knowledge.

Although intended as a book for the DCR student, other groups will find it useful, particularly candidates studying for the Higher Diploma of the College of Radiographers.

INTRODUCTION

The information included in this book is designed to assist the Diploma of the College of Radiographers (DCR) student in the study of osteology. My comments and advice are therefore directed toward student radiographers.

1 I would not claim that the book includes everything there is to know about the skeleton. If, for example, you wish to know more about the individual bones of the skull you should refer to one of the advanced anatomy books.

2 You have access to the skeleton and disarticulated bones. Get into the habit of looking at the bone as you study the relevant section. Identify the features mentioned in the text and talk to a tutor if you are unable to do so.

3 When you have completed each chapter look at old DCR examination papers, making sure that you could answer all relevant questions adequately.

4 Use your department experience. Get into the habit of testing your knowledge of radiographic anatomy on each radiograph you see and relate the position of tumours to specific features of the bone.

5 The pathology section in each chapter is for use as a guideline only. You can add to the list by taking an interest in the bony pathology you see in the departments.

6 The ossification section in each chapter includes dates of appearances and fusion of centres of ossification. You will not be tested on this in the DCR examination, but it is included so that you can learn to recognize ossification centres on radiographs of children and differentiate between epiphyseal lines and fractures.

7 The self-tests at the end of each chapter are included to enable you to assess your knowledge. You should complete the test without the use of the book and then check your answers. If you answer a question incorrectly, take time to look back at the chapter making sure you understand the correct answer.

ACKNOWLEDGEMENTS

I would like to acknowledge the help and advice given both by colleagues and students at Guy's Hospital during the preparation of this book. Special thanks to Miss M.E. Howard, Principal, Schools of Radiography and Radiotherapy, Guy's Hospital, and to Miss R.P. Klem and Miss Y.H. Yoe who have since moved on from Guy's. I would also like to thank Miss A. Baldrey, Principal, School of Therapeutic Radiography, Addenbrookes Hospital, Cambridge, for her very useful comments and suggestions. Finally, I would like to express my gratitude to my family for their support and, in particular, to my sister Mrs Gillian Rumsey and my niece Pippa for all their help in preparing the artwork and correcting the manuscript.

GLOSSARY

The terminology associated with bones may appear confusing at first glance but many terms are common to more than one bone. Given below is a short glossary to help you understand the meaning of the terms.

Projections and elevations

Condyle rounded process at the extremity of the bone, e.g. the condyles of the humerus.

Epicondyle projection of bone situated on a condyle, e.g. the epicondyles of the humerus.

Facet small, flat and smooth articular surface of a bone, e.g. the articular surface of a bone.

Process projection from the main body of a bone, e.g. the acromion process of the scapula.

Spine sharp, pointed, slender process, e.g. the spine of the scapula.

Trochanter protuberance of bone serving for the attachment of muscle, e.g. the greater trochanter of the femur.

Tubercle small, rounded projection, e.g. the tibial tubercle.

Tuberosity large, irregular projection of bone serving for attachment of muscle, e.g. the greater tuberosity of the humerus.

Depressions and holes

Foramen opening, hole or short passage, e.g. the obturator foramen of the hip bone.

Fossa shallow depression or pit, e.g. the olecranon fossa of the humerus.

Groove channel or furrow, e.g. the bicipital groove of the humerus.

Meatus tubular passage, e.g. the internal auditory meatus of the temporal bone.

The first bone to be described in Chapter 2 is a long bone consisting of a shaft and two extremities. The upper extremity bears a head and neck; this is the case in many bones. The term **head** simply means an expanded end of bone; the term **neck** means a constricted part connecting the head to the main mass of bone.

Before commencing your study of the bones ensure that you are thoroughly familiar with the standard anatomical position and the following related terms:

superior above, the upper of two parts;
inferior below, the lower of two parts;
medial towards the midline;
lateral away from the midline;
distal away from the centre of the body or point of origin;
proximal near to the centre of the body or point of origin;
anterior towards the front of the body;
posterior towards the back of the body.

CHAPTER 1
THE SKELETON

Osteology is the study of the bones and cartilages which make up the skeleton.

In the adult human body there are 206 bones which articulate together to form the skeleton.

The total of these 206 bones is formed thus:

Skull	22
Vertebral column	26
Ribs and sternum	25
Upper limb and shoulder girdle	64
Lower limb and pelvis	62
Auditory ossicles	6
Hyoid bone	1

THE STRUCTURE OF CARTILAGE (Fig. 1)

Classification

Cartilage is classified as a connective tissue but because of its solid consistency it is frequently regarded as a subdivision termed skeletal.

General description

Cartilage has particular features related to its function, e.g. it is rigid where it needs to bear weight. It may also be flexible but is always resilient to the stresses applied to it. The general structure is a group of cells situated within a matrix. The texture of the matrix governs the type of cartilage. There are three

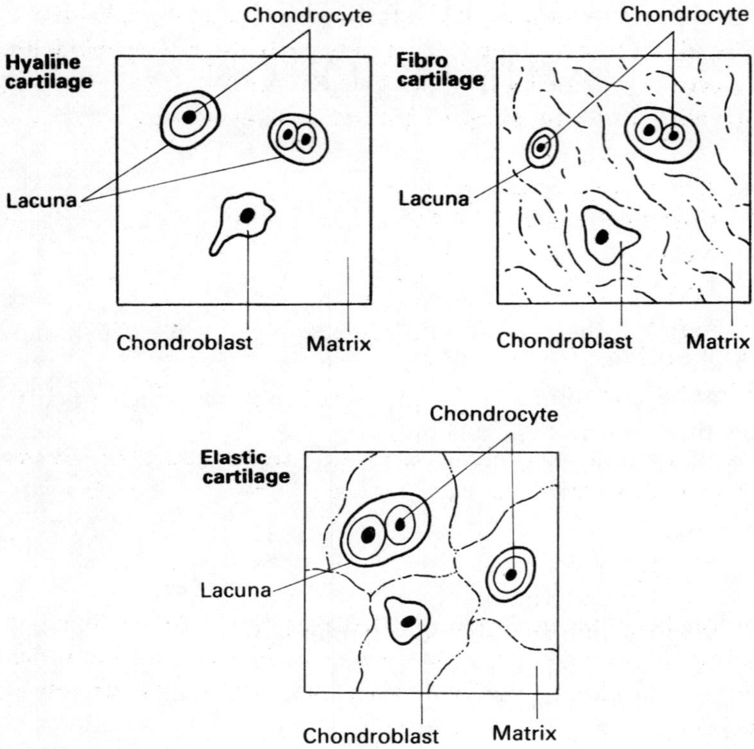

Fig. 1 The structure of cartilage.

types: hyaline, fibrous and elastic. There are two different types of cells within the matrix: chondrocytes and chondroblasts.

Chondrocytes usually have only a single nucleus which is round and central. The cytoplasm contains glycogen and lipid droplets. Chondrocytes are located within small spaces in the matrix termed lacunae.

Chondroblasts are precursors of chondrocytes. They are small, flattened cells, slightly irregular with surface projections.

Hyaline cartilage

Hyaline cartilage appears bluish white and glossy to look at. The matrix is even, with a ground substance like a firm gel consisting of mucopolysaccharide and mucoprotein. The matrix also has a 'feltwork' of fine, collagenous fibrils which are only visible with an electron microscope.

Hyaline cartilage is found at the following sites:

Articular cartilage
Costal cartilage
Nose
Larynx
Trachea
Bronchi
Bronchial tree

In addition to these sites in the body, hyaline cartilage forms embryonal cartilage, the precursor to the bony skeleton.

Fibrocartilage

Fibrocartilage has great strength and rigidity. The matrix has a ground substance identical to that of hyaline cartilage but it has many more collagenous fibrils which are visible with an optical microscope.

Fibrocartilage is found at the following sites:

Symphysis pubis
Intervertebral discs
Menisci of knee joint
Insertion of tendons, e.g. achilles tendon

Fibrocartilage also lines the grooves for the paths of tendons.

Elastic cartilage

Elastic cartilage has the ability to maintain its shape but also allows for some temporary change in shape.

The matrix has a ground substance as before but the network is of elastic fibres.

Elastic cartilage is found at the following sites:

Epiglottis
Some of the laryngeal cartilages
Pharyngo-tympanic tube
Pinna of ear

PERICHONDRIUM

Perichondrium is the membrane covering cartilage, except for articular surfaces of synovial joints which are smooth and bathed in synovial fluid to resist wear.

Structure

Perichondrium has two layers. The outer layer is white, fibrous tissue; the inner layer is vascular. This is important as cartilage has no direct blood supply and receives its nourishment from the perichondrium.

Functions

1 Nutrition as described above.
2 Repair process: in the event of damage to cartilage, perichondrial tissue invades the injured areas and is converted to cartilage.
3 Appositional growth (growth at the surface). Perichondrial cells can convert to chondroblasts and thence to chondrocytes to allow for appositional growth. Note: This is unlike cartilaginous interstitial growth (growth from within) which is due to the process of mitosis of the chondrocytes.

STRUCTURE OF BONE TISSUE

Classification

Bone tissue is classified as connective, skeletal tissue, i.e. the same as cartilage.

Features

Bone is vascular and constantly changing throughout life. The regenerative power of bone is good. It is hard and resilient, with tensile strength comparable to cast-iron, but with only one-third of its weight. The flexibility of bone tissue is comparable to that of steel, although it is not as strong.

General structure (Fig. 2)

Bone is similar to cartilage in that the general structure is one of cells within a matrix. The matrix is impregnated with mineral salts which makes it characteristically hard.

It is interesting to note that bone without mineral salts is so flexible that it is possible to tie a long bone into a knot! Bone without the organic matter is brittle and white and crumbles easily.

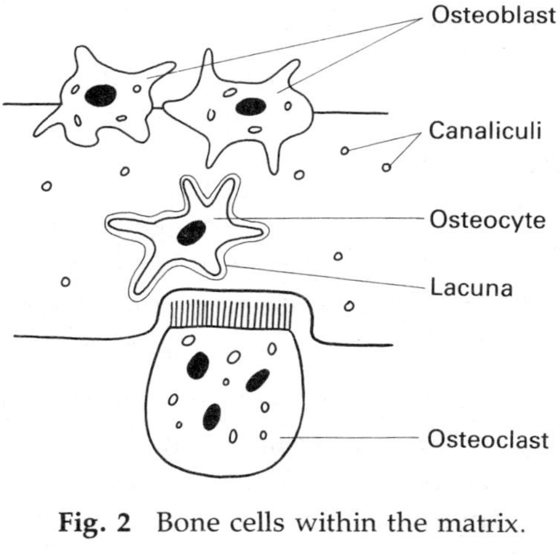

Fig. 2 Bone cells within the matrix.

Bone cells

Osteoblasts are situated on the surface of bone tissue. They are cuboidal in shape with cytoplasmic processes and organelles. The presence of organelles tells us that osteoblasts are very active cells. Their function is to secrete mucopolysaccharides, glycoprotein and proteins. These substances, with collagen fibres added, make up the osteoid tissue in which mineral salts are deposited.

Osteocytes develop from osteoblasts. They are considered to be 'captured' osteoblasts. They are situated within the matrix in small spaces called lacunae. The cytoplasmic processes project into canaliculi. The structure of osteocytes is similar to osteoblasts but the organelles are not so prominent, nor are there so many. It is thought that some cells have the same function as osteoblasts and that some have a different function, that of causing demineralization of surrounding tissue, thus increasing the size of the lacunae.

Osteoclasts are situated on the surface of growing tissue. They are giant cells with multiple nuclei and a brush border which is directed towards the matrix. They have many organelles, including phagocytotic vacuoles, lysosomes and mitochondria. Their function is to secrete substances able to break down mineral salts and collagen fibres so that the cell can phagocytose the remains.

Intercellular matrix

The organic matrix consists of many collagenous fibres with little ground substance. This ground substance consists of mucopolysaccharides, glycoproteins, serum proteins, water and electrolytes.

The mineral salts are inorganic salts which are mainly calcium phosphate and calcium carbonate, although other salts are present in smaller amounts. These include calcium fluoride, magnesium phosphate and sodium chloride. It is interesting to note that the calcium and phosphate ions situated on the surface of bone may enter the interstitial fluid and thus travel to the blood. There is therefore a constant interchange of salts between bone tissue and blood.

Macroscopic structure of bone

Macroscopically, bone may be considered to be either cancellous or compact. Cancellous bone consists of a meshwork of bone tissue and is spongy in appearance. Bone marrow is found in the many spaces. Cancellous bone is found at the extremities of long bones and in the middle of flat bones. Compact bone is dense and is formed into Haversian systems. This is the type of bone visible as a surround to all bones.

Microscopic structure of compact bone—the Haversian systems (Figs. 3–5)

Placed centrally to a Haversian system is a Haversian canal which contains an artery, vein and lymphatic vessel surrounded by a small amount of areolar tissue. Surrounding the Haversian canal are concentric rings of bone tissue called lamellae. Between the lamellae are fine, connecting channels called canaliculi. The lamellae have small spaces within the tissue called lacunae; these house the osteocytes. Haversian systems connect with one another by small channels called Volkmann's canals.

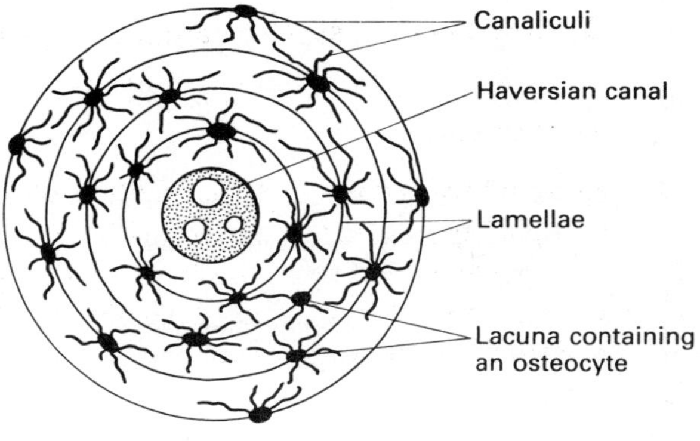

Fig. 3 Cross-section through Haversian system.

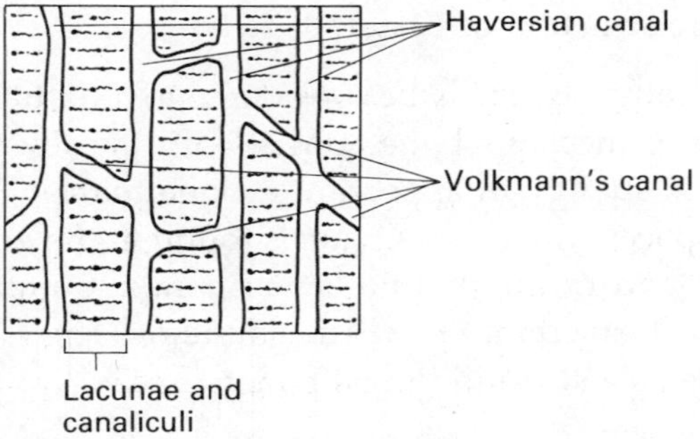

Fig. 4 Longitudinal section through bone to show several Haversian systems.

Figure 3 shows a cross-section through a Haversian system to show the features mentioned above.

Figure 4 shows a longitudinal section of several systems to show the oblique and transverse, connecting channels called Volkmann's canals.

Figure 5 shows several systems in a cross-sectional mode. The figure is much simplified and between the periosteum and medullary membrane of a long-bone shaft there would be many thousand Haversian systems. Between the Haversian systems are interstitial lamellae and encircling the inner and outer surfaces of the bone are circumferential lamellae.

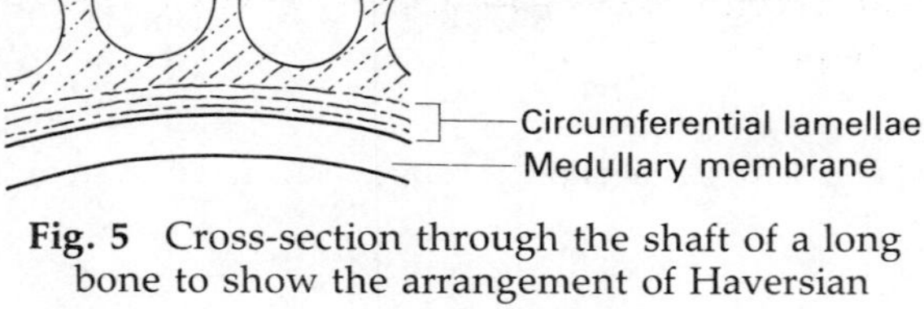

Fig. 5 Cross-section through the shaft of a long bone to show the arrangement of Haversian systems.

PERIOSTEUM

Periosteum covers bone except for the articular surfaces and at the attachment of tendons and ligaments where it blends with the outer covering of these structures. The outer layer of periosteum is white, fibrous tissue with some fat cells. The inner layer is a dense network of fine, elastic fibres. Separating this inner layer from bone is a layer of osteogenic tissue containing osteoblasts. It is from this tissue that appositional growth occurs (growth at surface). Periosteum is very vascular and the blood vessels communicate with those of the underlying bone.

BONE DEVELOPMENT AND GROWTH

Development of bone is either intramembranous (in membrane) or intracartilaginous (in cartilage). Most facial bones and bones of the skull vault develop from membrane and the rest develop from cartilage. The process of conversion into bone is called ossification.

Intramembranous development

Development of a bone of the skull vault

In early intrauterine life the brain is covered by three layers. The inner layer develops into the meninges, the outer layer develops into skin and the middle layer develops into bone and periosteum. This middle layer consists of fibres and osteoblasts. The osteoblasts lay down osteoid tissue into which mineral salts are deposited. The osteoblasts become captured and are then called osteocytes. In this way, successive layers of bone are deposited and compact bone is formed either side of the original cancellous bone.

Intracartilaginous development

Development of a long bone (Fig. 6)

In early intrauterine life buds of cartilage develop where the limbs are to be. A full cartilaginous skeleton is formed by the sixth week of intrauterine life.

Ossification begins at a primary centre termed the diaphysis. Initially, the cartilage cells in the centre enlarge and arrange themselves in rows. Mineral salts are deposited in the matrix which is produced by osteoblasts. The salts surround the cartilage cells which then die. Meanwhile, osteoclasts canalize the newly formed bone, making Haversian systems and the medullary cavity.

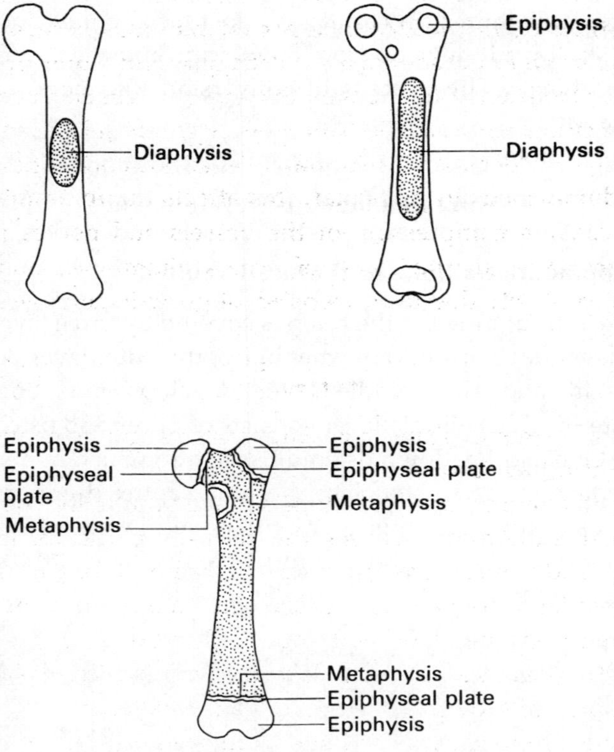

Fig. 6 Development of a long bone.

Most bones are formed from more than one centre of ossification. This secondary centre is called the epiphysis. The diaphysis and epiphysis are separated by a cartilaginous plate called the epiphyseal plate. At the extremity of the diaphysis is an area called the metaphysis; this is where growth in length of the bone occurs. At maturity, all the cartilage is converted to bone, the epiphyseal plate disappears and no more bone-growth occurs.

FACTORS CONTROLLING GROWTH

Diet

Calcium and phosphorus are essential for the normal growth of bone, as are vitamins D and C. Vitamin D is required for absorption of calcium from the gut. Vitamin C is necessary for the satisfactory production of collagen and mucopolysaccharide. Deficiency of vitamin D results in rickets; vitamin C deficiency causes scurvy. Vitamin A is required in small amounts. A deficiency of vitamin A causes osteoclastic activity to be diminished. In particular, this affects the foramina of the skull, causing compression of the vessels and nerves passing through them. In the event of excess vitamin A, bone pain occurs, probably due to the erosion of growth cartilage.

Hormones

Growth hormone is the most important of the hormones, but others also have an effect.

Parathormone and calcitonin have mutually opposing effects. Parathormone causes the release of calcium into the blood and oversecretion causes bone erosion and a demineralized framework. Calcitonin causes calcium to be extracted from the blood and deposited in bone.

Oestrogens increase osteoblastic activity, which explains the rapid spurt of growth which occurs after puberty.

Testosterone causes the bone to thicken with more calcium salts.

Thyroxin increases osteoclastic activity.

HEALING OF FRACTURES

Bone begins to heal as soon as a fracture occurs. The repair process is slightly different for compact and cancellous bone.

Repair of compact bone (Fig. 7)

During the injury, surrounding blood vessels tear and seep blood. In addition, periosteum and muscle is stripped from the bone.

A haematoma forms between and around the fractured surfaces. The haematoma is contained by soft tissues, i.e. the stripped periosteum and muscle.

The bone adjacent to the fracture site becomes ischaemic and bone cells die. This area of ischaemia is usually only a few millimetres in size.

The osteogenic tissue (containing osteoblasts) associated with the periosteum becomes active and forms a collar of tissue round the fracture fragments. As it develops it pushes the blood clot aside.

Simultaneously, there is an increased activity within the medullary cavity, with the endosteal cells forming a collar of tissue round the fracture fragments. In addition, the bone marrow begins to recover.

Both groups of cells (periosteal and endosteal) extend from one fracture fragment to the other. Within the growing tissue is a variable amount of cartilage.

The next stage is the formation of a callus. The cells mature to osteoblasts and chondroblasts. The osteoblasts produce the matrix into which the mineral salts are deposited. This newly formed, immature bone is sometimes referred to as woven bone. It forms a bridge which is radiologically visible. The fracture site is now rigid and secure.

Finally, the woven bone is gradually transformed to mature bone. The bone is strengthened and reshaped so that it is restored to its original form. A fracture with a bulbous callus will take a longer time to be restored. The size of the callus

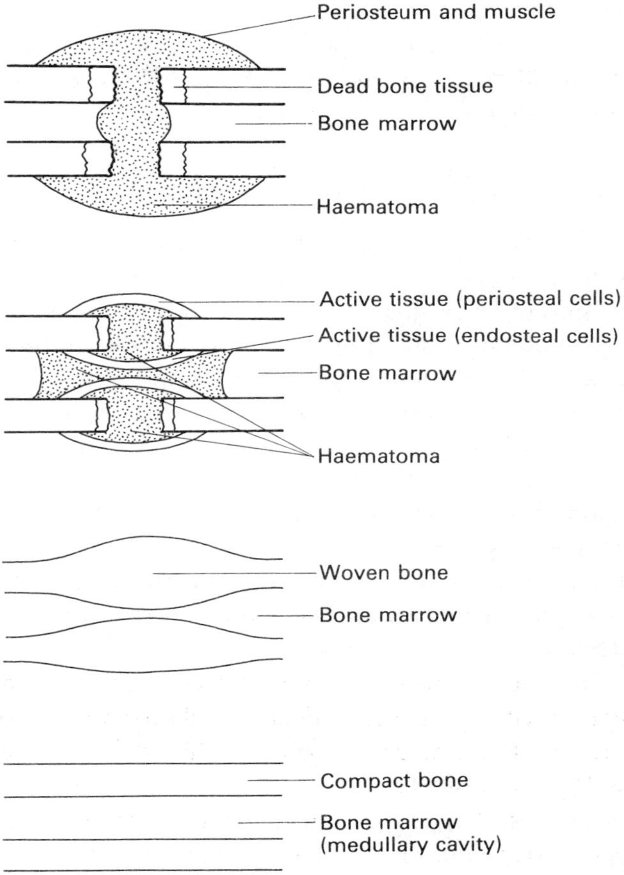

Fig. 7 Cross-section through a long bone to show the healing of compact bone.

depends on the amount of periosteal stripping, as well as the degree of displacement and the size of the haemotoma.

Repair of cancellous bone

Cancellous bone has no medullary cavity and therefore there is a broader area of contact. In addition, the meshwork allows for easier penetration of bone-forming tissue. Thus, healing is quicker compared to fractures of compact bone. The healing is by direct union, i.e. there is no stage of callus formation. Initially, a haematoma forms and is penetrated by blood vessels and proliferating osteogenic cells. A matrix is laid down and becomes ossified.

FUNCTIONS OF BONE

1 Protection, e.g. the brain is protected by the bones of the skull vault.
2 Provision of levers for muscles, thus permitting movement.
3 Support of soft tissue, therefore giving shape to the body.
4 Bones contain mineral salts and will permit substances to leave the bone and enter the blood stream in accordance with the body's needs, e.g. calcium ions may be taken from the bone if necessary.
5 Housing of bone marrow, important for blood-cell production.
6 Certain bones of the skull are pneumatic bones, i.e. they contain air. The function of these bones is to lighten the skull and add resonance to the voice.

CLASSIFICATION OF BONES

The bones of the skeleton are divided into five groups.

Long bones

Long bones consist of a shaft and two extremities. The shaft is compact bone surrounding a medullary cavity. The extremities are cancellous bone with a layer of compact. Examples of long bones are the femur, humerus and tibia. The clavicle, although classified as a long bone, does not possess a medullary cavity.

Short bones

Short bones are roughly cuboidal in shape. Although small, they possess great strength. The bone tissue is cancellous with a layer of compact. The tarsal bones are short bones, as are the carpal bones, except for the pisiform which is a sesamoid bone.

Flat bones

The function of flat bones is mainly protective. The bone tissue is like a sandwich formation with cancellous bone in the middle and compact bone either side. Examples of flat bones are the hip bone, bones of the skull vault and ribs.

Irregular bones

As the name suggests, irregular bones have no regular shape. The bone tissue is cancellous with a layer of compact. The vertebrae and the facial bones are examples of irregular bones.

Sesamoid bones

Sesamoid bones are unusual in that they develop in the tendons of muscles. The bone tissue is cancellous with a layer of compact. The patella and the pisiform are examples of sesamoid bones.

SELF–TEST

1 What is the classification of cartilage tissue?
2 Name the three types of cartilage.
3 Name two types of cartilage cells.
4 State the functions of perichondrium.
5 Name the three types of bone cells.
6 Name the two types of bone tissue visible to the human eye.
7 Name the structures transmitted in the Haversian canal.
8 What is meant by the terms diaphysis, epiphysis and metaphysis?
9 Name the substances necessary in the diet for satisfactory growth of bone.
10 Name the hormones affecting growth of bone tissue.
11 What is woven bone?

12 Classify the following bones:
Femur
Vertebrae
Tarsal bones
Ribs
Clavicle
Patella
Hip bone

Check your answers against those given at the back of the book.

CHAPTER 2
THE BONES OF THE UPPER LIMB

THE HUMERUS (Figs. 8 and 9)

Classification

The humerus is a long bone and therefore consists of an upper extremity, a shaft and a lower extremity.

Situation and articulations

The humerus is the bone of the upper arm. Superiorly it articulates with the glenoid cavity of the scapula to form the shoulder-joint. Inferiorly it articulates with the trochlear surface of the ulna and head of the radius to form the elbow-joint.

Bone tissue

The shaft is compact, surrounding a medullary cavity. The extremities are cancellous, surrounded by a thin layer of compact bone.

Description

The upper extremity

The *head* is described as being almost hemispherical. It is directed superiorly, medially and slightly posteriorly to articulate with the glenoid cavity of the scapula.

The *anatomical neck* is a slight constriction separating the head of the humerus from the tuberosities.

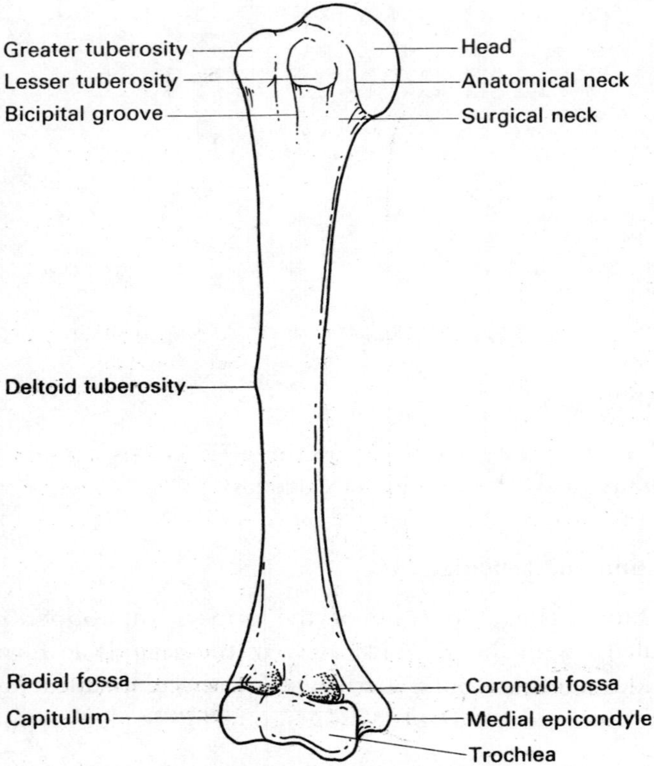

Fig. 8 Right humerus — anterior aspect.

The *greater tuberosity* is situated on the lateral aspect of the upper extremity. It has three impressions for the insertion of three muscles; the supraspinatus, infraspinatus and teres minor.

The *lesser tuberosity* is the smaller of the two tuberosities, situated on the anterior aspect of the upper extremity. It gives attachment to the subscapularis muscle.

The *bicipital groove* is a well-defined ridge situated between the tuberosities. The tendon of the long head of biceps runs in this groove. The margins of the bicipital groove also give attachment to several other muscles; the pectoralis major, teres minor and latissimus dorsi.

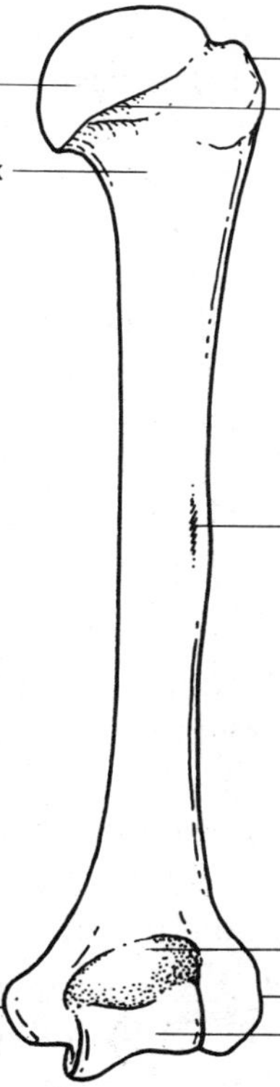

Fig. 9 Right humerus — posterior aspect.

The *surgical neck* separates the upper extremity from the shaft. It is a common site of fracture. The axillary nerve and the posterior humeral circumflex artery are in close proximity to it.

The shaft

The upper half of the shaft is almost cylindrical, becoming triangular as it is flattened from front to back at its lower portion.

The shaft is described as having three surfaces and three borders, although the boundaries of these are not altogether clear. The lateral border is crossed by the spiral groove in which the radial nerve runs. The antero-lateral surface bears the deltoid tuberosity which takes the attachment of the deltoid muscle. The antero-medial surface usually bears the nutrient foramen.

The lower extremity

The *medial and lateral condyles* are each surmounted by epicondyles. The condyles are formed by the side-to-side expansion of the lower extremity. The medial epicondyle is prominent and easily palpable; the ulnar nerve is in close proximity. Extending superiorly from the epicondyles are ridges: the medial and lateral supracondylar ridges.

The *trochlea* is the medial of the two articular surfaces. It extends from the front to back of the humerus and is lipped, the medial lip being the larger. It is sometimes described as being pulley shaped. It articulates with the trochlear notch of the ulna. Because of its lipped nature, when the arm is extended the angle between the lateral border of the humerus and the radius is less than 180°. This is the carrying angle and is necessary in order for the arms to swing clear of the hips. The carrying angle is therefore more marked in females than males.

The *capitulum* is lateral to the trochlea. It is a rounded, convex, anterior, articular surface which articulates with the head of the radius.

The olecranon fossa is an oval hollow situated on the posterior part of the lower extremity, above the trochlea. It accommodates the olecranon process of the ulna when the arm is extended.

The *radial fossa* is the lateral of the two anterior fossae of the humerus. It is situated above the capitulum and accommodates the head of the radius when the arm is flexed.

The *coronoid fossa* is medial to the radial fossa. It accommodates the coronoid process of the ulna when the arm is flexed.

Blood supply

The brachial artery drains to the brachial vein.

Nerve supply

The brachial nerve.

Ossification

The humerus is ossified from eight centres:

The shaft appears at the eighth week of intrauterine life.
The head appears six months after birth.
The greater tuberosity appears in the second year.
The lesser tuberosity appears in the fifth year.

The head, greater and lesser tuberosities unite in the sixth to seventh year and join the shaft in the twentieth year.

The capitulum and lateral part of the trochlea appear in the first year.
The medial part of the trochlea appears in the ninth year.
The lateral epicondyle appears in the twelfth year.

The capitulum, lateral and medial part of the trochlea and the lateral epicondyle unite in the fourteenth year in females and in the sixteenth year in males.

The medial epicondyle appears between the fourth and sixth year and unites with the rest of the bone in the twentieth year.

Pathology

Fractures of the humerus frequently endanger structures, e.g. medial epicondyle fracture may involve the ulnar nerve and a supracondylar fracture may involve the brachial artery and/or the median nerve. A fracture of the surgical neck may involve the circumflex nerve.

Calcareous tendinitis is calcification of the sheaths of tendons. It most frequently occurs near the insertion of the supraspinatus tendon, but may also occur at the insertion of the infraspinatus or the biceps tendon.

Secondary deposits may occur in the humerus, the primary tumour usually being in the breast or lungs.

THE ULNA (Figs. 10 and 11)

Classification

The ulna is classified as a long bone.

Situation and articulations

The ulna is the medial bone of the forearm. It articulates at its upper end with the trochlea of the humerus, forming part of the elbow-joint, and with the head of the radius, forming the superior radioulnar joint. At its lower end, the ulna is in contact with an articular disc which forms part of the wrist-joint and with the ulnar notch of the radius, forming the inferior radioulnar joint.

Bone tissue

The shaft of the ulna is compact bone surrounding a medullary cavity. The extremities are cancellous with a layer of compact bone.

Description

The upper extremity

The *olecranon process* forms the uppermost part of the ulna. Its upper border forms the point of the elbow. The posterior surface is palpable. The anterior surface is smooth and forms the upper part of the trochlear notch. The olecranon process is accommodated in the olecranon fossa of the humerus when the arm is extended.

The *coronoid process* is the anterior projection immediately below the olecranon process. The upper surface is smooth and forms

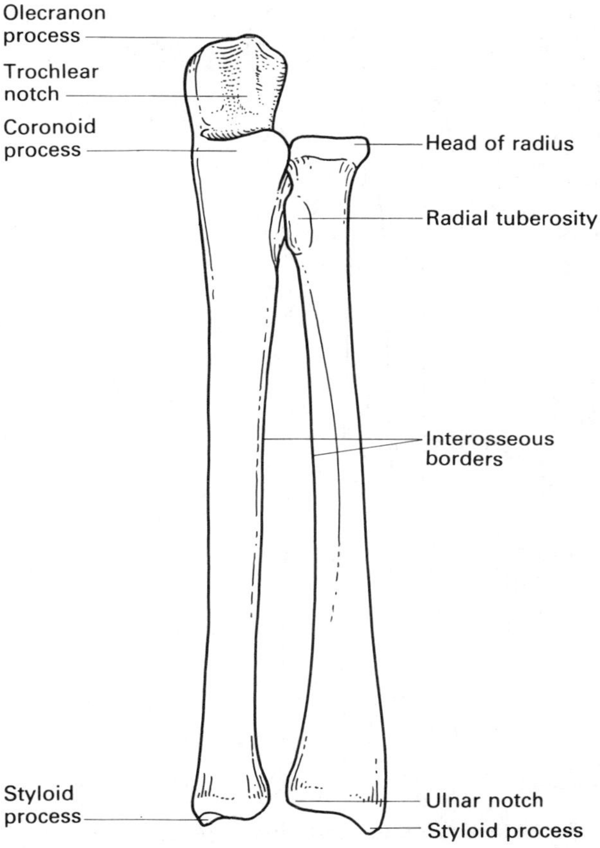

Fig. 10 Left radius and ulna — anterior aspect.

the lower part of the trochlear notch. The coronoid process is accommodated in the coronoid fossa of the humerus when the arm is flexed.

The *radial notch* is situated on the lateral surface of the upper extremity. It articulates with the circumference of the head of the radius. Below the notch is an indentation which accommodates the radial tuberosity of the radius during rotational movements of the forearm.

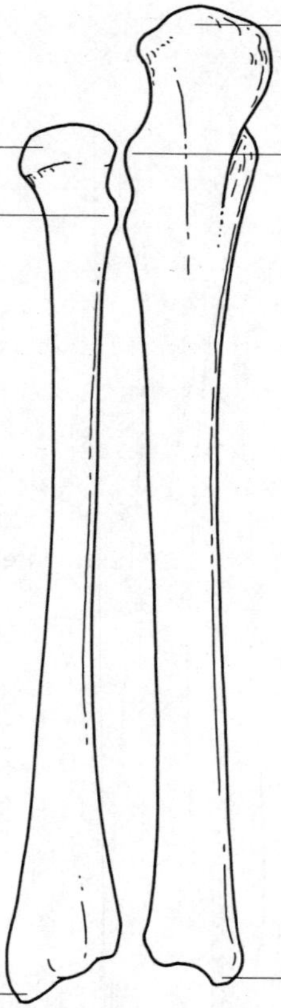

Fig. 11 Left radius and ulna — posterior aspect.

A *tuberosity* is situated inferior to the coronoid process on the anterior surface of the upper extremity. It gives attachment to the brachialis muscle.

The *trochlear notch* articulates with the trochlea of the humerus. A smooth ridge divides the trochlear notch into a medial and a smaller lateral surface.

The shaft

The shaft of the ulna is triangular in cross-section above, becoming almost cylindrical at its lower end. The lateral border is the interosseous border and gives attachment to the interosseous membrane. The anterior surface usually bears the nutrient foramen.

The lower extremity

The *head* presents a convex, articular surface for the ulnar notch of the radius, forming the inferior radioulnar joint. The inferior surface is smooth and is separated from the carpal bones by an articular disc.

The *styloid process* is a projection of the postero-medial aspect of the ulna. It is easily palpable.

Blood supply

The ulnar artery drains to the ulnar vein.

Nerve supply

The ulnar nerve.

Ossification

The shaft appears at approximately the eighth week of intrauterine life.
The lower extremity appears in the fifth year in females and sixth year in males.
These unite with the shaft in the seventeenth year in females and eighteenth year in males.
The upper extremity appears in the ninth year in females and eleventh year in males and unites with the shaft in the fourteenth year in females and sixteenth year in males.

Pathology

See the pathology of the radius.

THE RADIUS (Figs. 10 and 11)

Classification

The radius is classified as a long bone.

Situation and articulations

The radius is the lateral bone of the forearm. It articulates at its upper end with the capitulum of the humerus, forming part of the elbow joint, and with the radial notch of the ulna, forming the superior radioulnar joint. At its lower end the radius articulates with the scaphoid and lunate bones to form part of the wrist-joint, and with the ulna, to form the inferior radioulnar joint.

Bone tissue

The shaft of the radius is compact surrounding a medullary cavity. The extremities are cancellous with a layer of compact bone.

Description

The upper extremity

The *head* of the radius is disc shaped. The superior surface is concave to articulate with the capitulum. The circumference articulates with the radial notch of the ulna.

The *neck* is a slight constriction below the head.

The *radial tuberosity* situated below the neck gives attachment to the biceps tendon.

The shaft

The shaft of the radius is triangular in cross-section. The medial border is sharp and is the interosseous border which gives attachment to the interosseous membrane. The anterior surface usually bears the nutrient foramen.

The lower extremity

The *styloid process* is a projection of the lateral surface. This process is easily palpable.

The *inferior surface* is smooth and articulates with the lunate and scaphoid, forming part of the wrist-joint.

The *ulnar notch* is located on the medial surface. It articulates with the head of the ulna, forming the inferior radioulnar joint.

Blood supply

The radial artery drains to the radial vein.

Nerve supply

The radial nerve.

Ossification

The shaft appears in the eighth week of intrauterine life. The lower extremity appears at the end of the first year of life and fuses with the shaft at seventeen years in females and nineteen years in males. The upper extremity appears in the fourth year in females and fifth year in males and fuses with the shaft in the fourteenth year in females and seventeenth year in males.

Pathology (radius and ulna)

A *Colles' fracture* is a fracture of the radius approximately 2–3 cm proximal to the wrist-joint, the distal fragment being displaced posteriorly.

A *Galeazzi fracture* is a fracture of the radius associated with a dislocation of the distal extremity of the ulna.

A *Monteggia fracture* is a fracture of the upper shaft of the ulna associated with a dislocation of the head of the radius.

THE HAND (Fig. 12)

The hand is composed of three groups of bones: the phalanges, the metacarpals and the carpal bones.

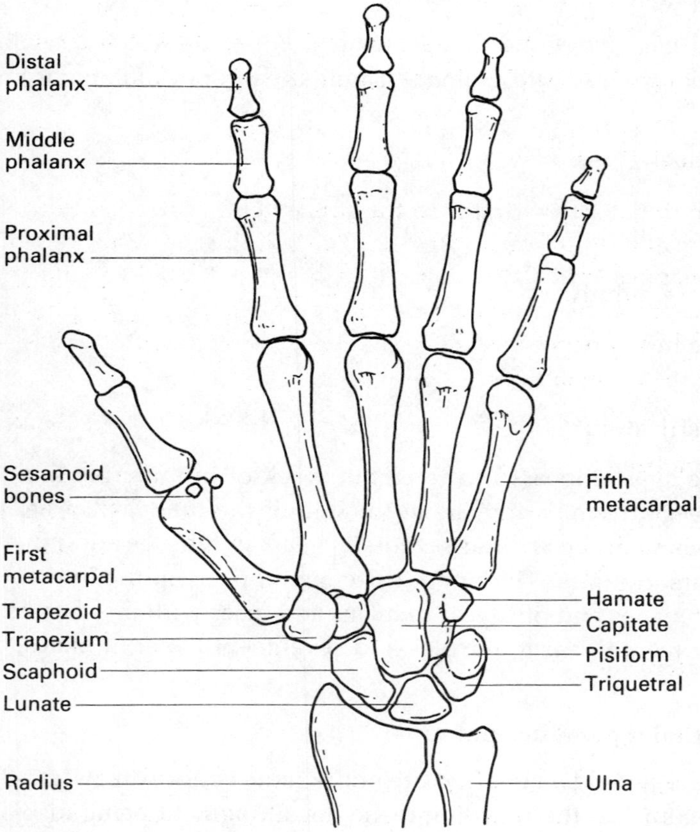

Fig. 12 Left hand — palmar aspect.

The phalanges

The phalanges of the hand are similar in number and arrangement to those of the foot.

The thumb has two phalanges: the distal and proximal. The other four fingers have three: the distal, middle and proximal.

Classification

The phalanges are long bones and therefore consist of a shaft and two extremities. The proximal extremity is known as the base and the distal extremity as the head.

Articulations

The bases of the proximal phalanges articulate with the corresponding metacarpals. The heads of the proximal phalanges articulate with the bases of the middle phalanges (except for the thumb which, of course, has no middle phalanx). The heads of the middle phalanges articulate with the bases of the distal phalanges.

Bone tissue

The shaft is compact bone surrounding a medullary cavity. The extremities are cancellous, surrounded by a thin layer of compact bone.

Description

The proximal phalanges

The shafts of the proximal phalanges are convex dorsally and concave on the palmar aspect. The base of each presents an oval, concave facet for articulation with the appropriate head of a metacarpal. The head presents a facet for articulation with the middle phalanx.

The middle phalanges

The middle phalanges are shorter and smaller than the proximal phalanges.

The distal phalanges

The bases of the distal phalanges articulate with the heads of the middle phalanges. The heads are expanded to support the pulp of the finger tips.

The metacarpals

The five metacarpal bones connect the carpal bones to the phalanges, forming the bony framework of the hand. They are numbered one to five from the lateral side.

Classification

The metacarpals are long bones. They therefore consist of a shaft and two extremities. The proximal extremity is known as the base and the distal extremity as the head.

Articulations

The heads of the metacarpals articulate with the bases of the proximal phalanges of the corresponding fingers.

The bases of the metacarpals articulate as follows.

The first metacarpal articulates with the trapezium.
The second metacarpal articulates with the third metacarpal, trapezium, trapezoid and capitate.
The third metacarpal articulates with the second metacarpal, fourth metacarpal and capitate.
The fourth metacarpal articulates with the third metacarpal, fifth metacarpal, capitate and hamate.
The fifth metacarpal articulates with the fourth metacarpal and hamate.

Bone tissues

The shaft is compact surrounding a medullary cavity. The extremities are cancellous with a layer of compact bone.

Description

The first metacarpal is short and thick. It lies obliquely, forming a synovial saddle joint with the trapezium. The shape of the first metacarpal and the saddle joint permits a grasping movement. Sesamoid bones are present at the site of the first metacarpo-carpal joint. The second, third, fourth and fifth metacarpals have rounded heads to articulate with the phalanges, forming the metacarpo-phalangeal joints. The bases articulate with the carpal bones and with each other.

The carpal bones

The carpal bones consist of eight bones arranged in two rows of four. The proximal row consists of the scaphoid, lunate, triquetral and pisiform. The distal row consists of the trapezium, trapezoid, capitate and hamate.

Classification

The carpal bones are short bones, except for the pisiform which is a sesamoid bone.

Articulations

The scaphoid articulates with the radius, capitate, lunate, trapezium and trapezoid.
The lunate articulates with the radius, capitate, scaphoid and triquetral.
The triquetral articulates with the articular disc of the ulna, pisiform, lunate and hamate.
The pisiform articulates with the triquetral.
The trapezium articulates with the first metacarpal, second

metacarpal, trapezoid and scaphoid.
The trapezoid articulates with the second metacarpal, capitate, trapezium and scaphoid.
The capitate articulates with the second metacarpal, third metacarpal, fourth metacarpal, scaphoid, lunate, trapezoid and hamate.
The hamate articulates with the fourth metacarpal, fifth metacarpal, lunate, triquetral and capitate.

Bone tissue

The carpal bones are cancellous bone with a layer of compact.

Description

The scaphoid

The scaphoid is the largest of the proximal carpals. It is described as being boat shaped. The palmar surface presents a prominent tubercle.

The lunate

The lunate is so called because it is crescentic in shape.

The triquetral

The triquetral is wedge shaped.

The pisiform

The pisiform is a sesamoid bone. It is small and spherical in shape.

The trapezium

The trapezium is cuboidal and the lateral surface bears a tubercle.

The trapezoid

The trapezoid is a small, irregularly shaped bone.

The capitate

The capitate is the largest of the carpal bones. The proximal surface is convex for articulation with the scaphoid and lunate and is termed the head of the capitate.

The hamate

The hamate is wedge shaped with a projection on the palmar surface called the hook of hamate.

The palmar arch

The carpal bones form an arch, concave anteriorly. Its prominence is increased by the tubercle of the trapezium, hook of hamate, tubercle of scaphoid and pisiform. Enclosing the arch, forming a tunnel, is a ligament — the flexor retinaculum. Through the arch passes blood and nerve supplies to the hand.

Essential aspects of the hand

Blood supply

The hand is supplied by the palmar arch, which is formed by an anastomosis of the radial and ulnar arteries. Blood drains to tributaries of the radial and ulnar veins.

Nerve supply

Branches of the ulnar, radial and median nerves are responsible for innervation of the hand.

Ossification

The carpal bones each develop from a single centre. The capitate and hamate appear in the first year of life. The triquetral appears in the third year. The trapezium and lunate appear in the fifth year, the scaphoid in the sixth year, the trapezoid in the eighth year and finally the pisiform appears in the twelfth year.

The metacarpals develop from two centres each. The shaft appears in the eighth week of life. The distal extremity of the second, third, fourth and fifth metacarpals and the proximal extremity of the first metacarpal appear in the third year and unite with the shaft in the twentieth year.

The shaft of each phalanx appears in the eighth week and the proximal extremity appears in the fourth year, uniting with the shaft between the eighteenth and twentieth years.

Pathology

Fractures of the hand are common, especially the following:

- Crush fractures of the distal phlanges
- Fracture of the fifth metacarpal
- Fracture of the scaphoid following a fall on the outstretched hand (the blood supply of the scaphoid is frequently effected, making healing of this bone difficult)
- Bennetts fracture, the name given to a fracture of the base of the first metacarpal

Keinbock's disease is osteochondritis of the lunate bone.

Rheumatoid arthritis frequently presents in the small joints of the hand, e.g. the metacarpo-phalangeal joints.

Hyperparathyroidism is an endocrine disorder which causes erosion of bone tissue. Radiography of the hand may be requested for diagnosis of this disease. Erosion of the necks of the metacarpals and/or the terminal phalanges is indicative of hyperparathyroidism.

Carpal tunnel syndrome occurs due to compression of the median nerve within the carpal tunnel. It may be due to arthritic changes or bony injury. The symptoms are paraesthesia, numbness and motor weakness.

SELF–TEST

1 Classify the humerus.
2 List the articulations of the humerus.
3 Distinguish between the anatomical and surgical necks of the humerus.
4 Which tendon runs in the bicipital groove?
5 Name the three fossae of the lower extremity of the humerus.
6 State the bone tissue of the ulna.
7 Name the two processes of the upper extremity of the ulna.
8 Which border of the ulna is the interosseus border?
9 Which is the lateral bone of the forearm?
10 Which carpal bones articulate with the radius?
11 Classify the phalanges.
12 Name the type of joint formed between the first metacarpal and trapezium.
13 List the carpal bones in the distal row.
14 What is Keinbock's disease?

Check your answers against those given at the back of the book.

CHAPTER 3
THE BONES OF THE SHOULDER GIRDLE

THE SCAPULA (Figs. 13 and 14)

Classification

The scapula is classified as a flat bone.

Situation and articulations

The scapula is a flat, triangular bone forming part of the shoulder girdle. It is superficial and easily palpable. It is situated on the posterior thoracic wall, extending from the level of the second rib to that of the seventh. The glenoid cavity of the scapula articulates with the head of the humerus, forming the shoulder joint. The acromion process of the scapula articulates with the clavicle, forming the acromioclavicular joint.

Bone tissue

The scapula consists of cancellous bone in the processes, lateral angle and lateral border. Surrounding these and elsewhere is compact bone.

Description

Since the scapula is flat and triangular, it consists of two surfaces, three borders and three angles. It also has two processes and a spine.

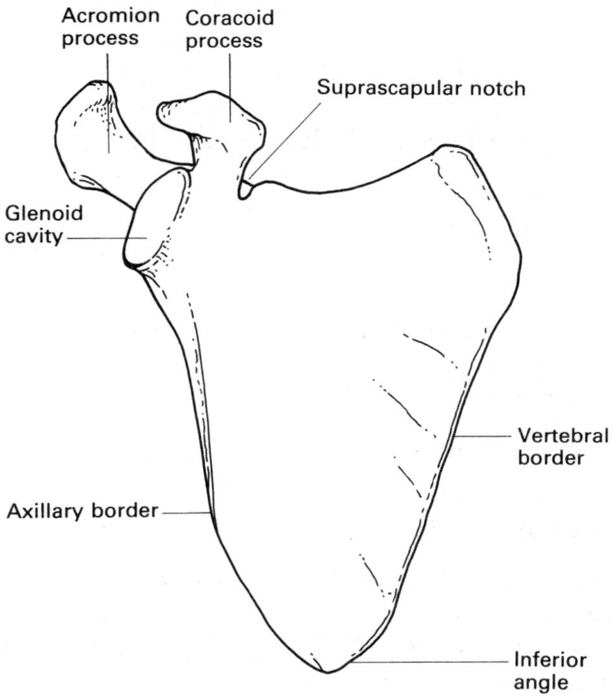

Fig. 13 Right scapula — anterior aspect.

The surfaces

The *anterior or costal surface* is slightly concave, allowing for the curvature of the posterior thoracic wall. This surface gives attachment to the origin of the subscapularis muscle.

The *posterior or dorsal surface* is crossed by the spine which divides the surface into two fossae: the supraspinous fossa and the infraspinous fossa. The two fossae are linked by the spinoglenoid notch. The supraspinous fossa gives attachment to the origin of the supraspinatus muscle and the infraspinous fossa gives attachment to the origin of the infraspinatus muscle.

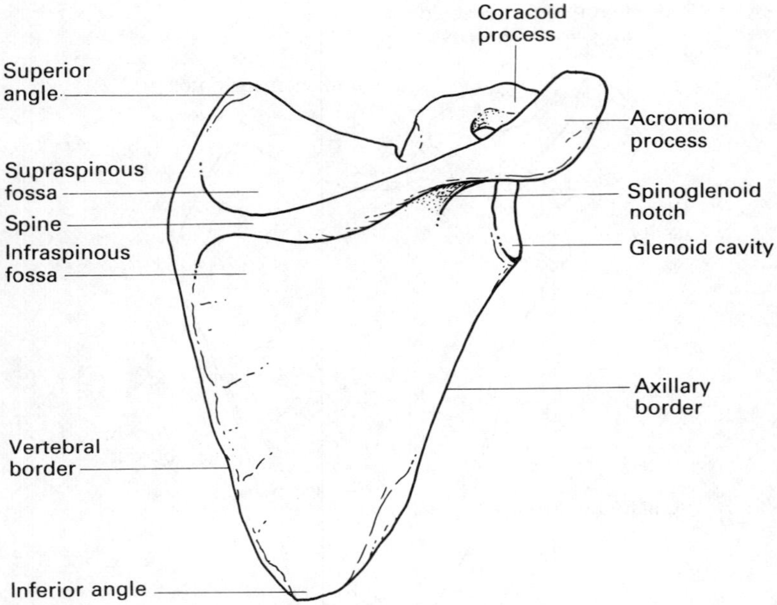

Fig. 14 Right scapula — posterior aspect.

The borders

The *superior border* is the shortest of the three borders. It ends laterally in the suprascapular notch and coracoid process.

The *medial or vertebral border* is very superficial. This border is parallel to the vertebrae when the arm is by the side.

The *lateral or axillary border* extends from the glenoid cavity to the inferior angle. This border is thicker than the rest and gives attachment to the teres minor, teres major and the long head of triceps muscle.

The angles

The *superior angle* is situated between the superior and medial borders.

The *inferior angle* is situated between the medial and lateral borders.

The *lateral angle* is thick and is sometimes called the head of the scapula. It has a short neck connecting it to the glenoid cavity. The glenoid cavity is a shallow, pear-shaped, concave depression which articulates with the head of the humerus. The glenoid cavity is deepened by a rim of cartilage.

The spine

The spine is a shelf of bone extending across the posterior surface from the medial border. It becomes continuous with the acromion process. It gives attachment to the origin of the deltoid muscle.

The processes

The *coracoid process* projects forwards and outwards to overhang the shoulder joint. It gives attachment to the short head of biceps and the coracobrachialis muscle.

The *acromion process* is a flattened, oblong, lateral projection of the spine and is situated at right angles to it. Medially, it has a facet for articulation with the clavicle. It gives attachment to the origin of the deltoid muscle.

Blood supply

The axillary artery drains to the axillary vein.

Nerve supply

The axillary nerve.

Ossification

Ossification of the scapula occurs from eight centres, sometimes more. The body appears at the eighth week of intrauterine life. The middle of the coracoid process appears in the first year and unites with the body in the fifteenth year. The rest of the coracoid process, rim of the lower part of the glenoid cavity, acromion process (two centres), inferior angle and medial border all appear at puberty and join the body by the twentieth year.

Pathology

Although the scapula is superficial, *fractures* of the scapula are uncommon. This is because of the protective muscle surround.

Os acromiale is a developmental anomaly whereby the acromion process does not unite with the rest of the scapula.

Sprengel's deformity is a congenital deformity producing an elevated scapula which may be united with the cervical vertebrae.

THE CLAVICLE (Fig. 15)

Classification

The clavicle is a long bone.

Situation and articulations

The clavicle extends almost horizontally across the root of the neck. It is superficial and easily palpable along its entire length. It articulates with the acromion process of the scapula, forming the acromioclavicular joint, and with the clavicular notch of the manubrium sterni and the first costal cartilage, forming the sternoclavicular joint. The function of the clavicle is to aid in holding the shoulder joint out laterally.

Bone tissue

Although the clavicle is a long bone it is unusual in that it possesses no medullary cavity. This is because the clavicle ossifies from a mixture of membrane and cartilage. The bone tissue is cancellous with a layer of compact.

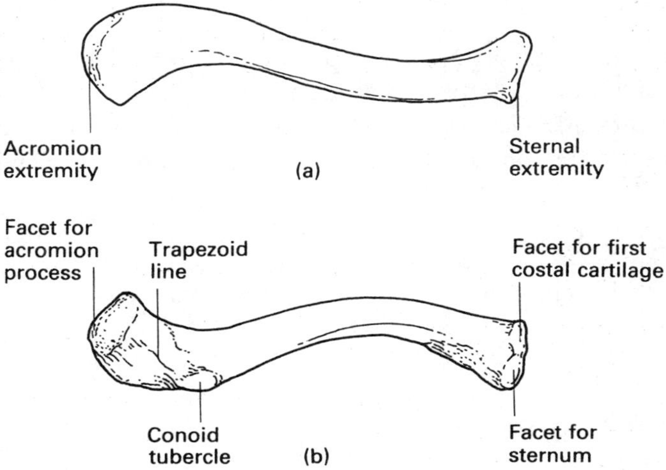

Fig. 15 Right clavicle — superior (a) and inferior (b) aspects.

Description

The clavicle consists of a shaft and two extremities.

The acromion extremity

The acromion extremity is flattened into superior and inferior surfaces. The anterior border gives attachment to the origin of the deltoid muscle. The acromion end presents an oval facet for the articulation with the acromion process of the scapula, forming the acromioclavicular joint.

The shaft

The shaft presents two curves. The medial two-thirds is convex, forward and rounded. The lateral third is concave, forward and flattened. The inferolateral surface bears the conoid tubercle for attachment of the coracoclavicular ligament. This surface also bears the trapezoid line which takes the insertion of a ligament of the trapezius muscle.

The sternal extremity

The sternal extremity is thick and chunky. It articulates with the clavicular notch of the manubrium sterni and with the first costal cartilage via two facets. The costoclavicular ligament is attached to the inferior surface of the sternal end of the clavicle.

Blood supply

The subclavian artery drains to the subclavian vein.

Nerve supply

The axillary nerve.

Ossification

The clavicle is the first bone of the skeleton to ossify. The shaft ossifies from two primary centres which appear at the fifth to sixth week of intrauterine life and fuse at six to seven weeks. The sternal and acromial ends appear at approximately the nineteenth to twenty-second year and unite quickly with the rest of the shaft.

Pathology

Fractures of the clavicle are common and are often due to indirect trauma. The commonest fracture site is at the junction of the lateral third to the medial two-thirds.

SELF TEST

1 List the articulations of the scapula.
2 State the situation of the scapula.
3 Name the structure which divides the posterior surface of the scapula.
4 Describe the shape of the glenoid cavity.
5 Name the three angles of the scapula.

6 Which process of the scapula gives attachment to the short head of the biceps?
7 What is unusual about the bone tissue of the clavicle?
8 What is the name given to the medial end of the clavicle?
9 What is the name given to the lateral end of the clavicle?
10 Name the articulations of the medial end of the clavicle.

Check your answers against those given at the back of the book.

CHAPTER 4
THE BONES OF THE LOWER LIMB

THE FEMUR (Figs. 16–18)

Classification

The femur is a long bone and therefore consists of an upper extremity, a shaft and a lower extremity.

Situation and articulations

The femur is the thigh bone. It is the longest and heaviest bone of the skeleton. Superiorly it articulates with the acetabulum of the hip bone to form the hip-joint. Inferiorly it articulates with the posterior surface of the patella and the condyles of the tibia to form the knee-joint. In the erect position, the femora are directed medially so that superiorly the heads are separated by the width of the pelvis, but inferiorly the medial condyles touch at the knee. This degree of inclination is greater in the female than the male.

Bone tissue

The shaft consists of compact bone surrounding a medullary cavity. The extemities are cancellous, surrounded by a thin layer of compact bone.

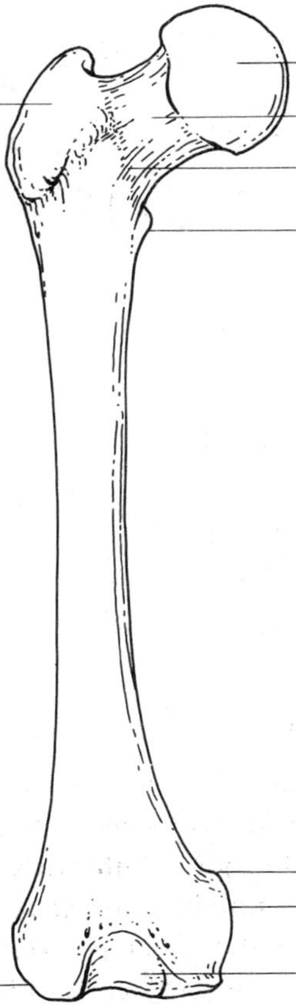

Fig. 16 Right femur — anterior aspect.

Description

The upper extremity

The *head* is described as being two-thirds of a sphere. It is directed superiorly, medially and slightly anteriorly to articulate with the acetabulum of the hip bone. The head is smooth except for a shallow, rough depression just below its centre. This is called the fovea and gives attachment to the ligament of the head of the femur.

The *neck* is a thick bar approximately 5 cm long in the adult. It is flattened from front to back, presenting superior and inferior borders. The superior border is short and gently concave upwards. The inferior border is longer and oblique and joins the shaft near the lesser trochanter. The neck joins the head to the shaft at an angle of approximately 125°; this allows for clearance of the pelvis by the femur. This angle is less in the female than the male.

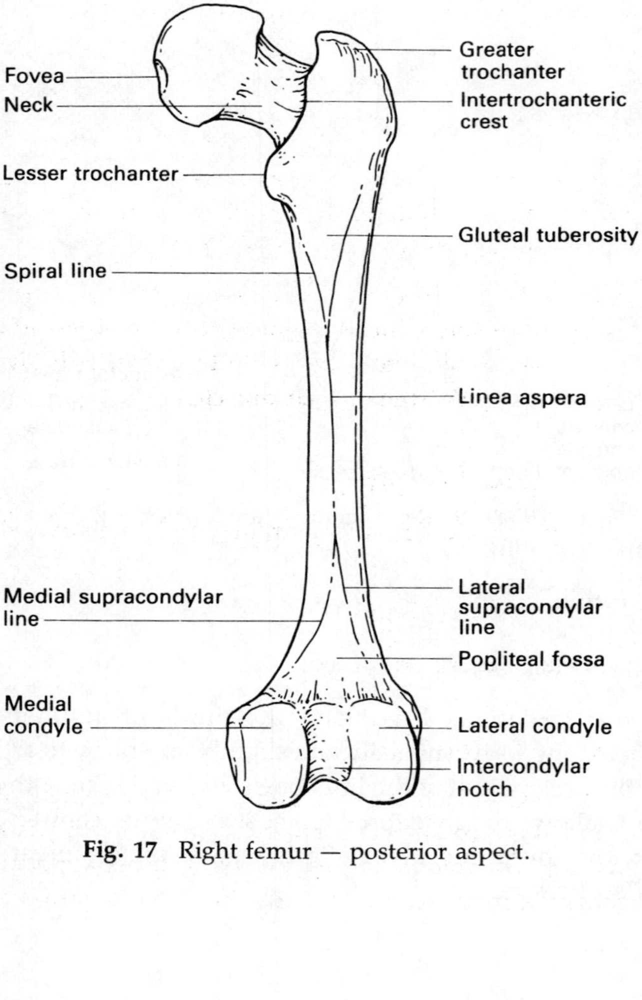

Fig. 17 Right femur — posterior aspect.

The *greater trochanter* is easily palpable. It projects superiorly from the point where the neck meets the shaft and gives attachment to most of the muscles of the gluteal region.

The *lesser trochanter* is conical in shape and projects postero-medially. Its muscle attachments include the psoas major muscle.

The *intertrochanteric line* is a rough ridge which runs anteriorly over the surface of the neck, between the two trochanters.

The *intertrochanteric crest* is a well-marked, rounded ridge which runs posteriorly between the two trochanters.

The *trochanteric fossa* lies posteriorly and is overhung by the greater trochanter.

The shaft

The shaft is roughly cylindrical in cross-section. It is narrowest at its middle, expanding above and below. The anterior surface is slightly convex, the posterior surface slightly concave.

The *linea aspera* extends as a ridge down the posterior surface of the femoral shaft. At the junction of the middle-third with the lower-third of the shaft the linea aspera divides again, forming the medial and lateral supracondylar lines.

The *gluteal tuberosity* is a roughened ridge which extends upwards and laterally to the greater trochanter. It is continuous below with the lateral lip of the linea aspera.

The *spiral line* is continuous above with the lower part of the intertrochanteric line and below with the medial lip of the linea aspera.

The *popliteal fossa* is a triangular-shaped area on the posterior surface of the shaft. It is formed by the diverging medial and lateral supracondylar lines.

Nutrient foramina of which there are usually two, are located close to the linea aspera.

The lower extremity

The lower extremity is expanded into two large condyles, thus providing a large area for weight transference.

The *lateral condyle* is the smaller of the two condyles. It has extensive anterior, posterior and inferior articular surfaces, forming part of the knee-joint. It is surmounted by an epicondyle.

The *medial condyle* also has extensive articular surfaces. The uppermost part of the medial condyle bears the adductor tubercle, so called because it gives attachment to the tendon of the adductor magnus muscle. The medial condyle is also surmounted by an epicondyle.

The *intercondylar notch* is a deep, posterior groove, which is formed by the backward projection of the condyles.

The *patellar surface* is a shallow fossa formed anteriorly by the union of the condyles. It extends superiorly more on the lateral side than the medial. It is this surface with which the patella articulates.

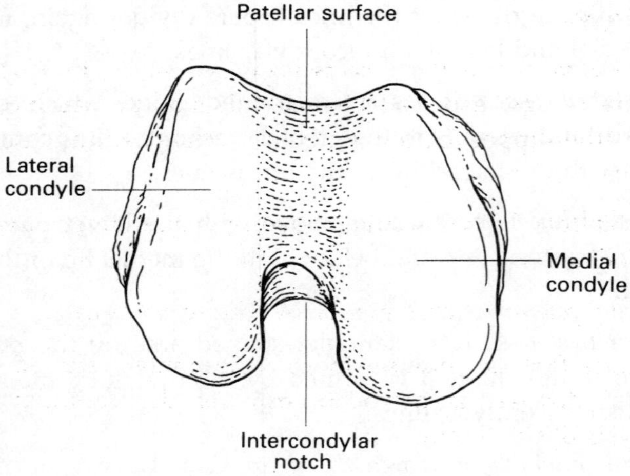

Fig. 18 Right femur — inferior aspect of the lower extremity.

Blood supply

The femoral artery drains to the femoral vein.

Nerve supply

The femoral nerve.

Ossification

The shaft appears at the seventh week of intrauterine life.
The head appears at six months and fuses to the shaft in the eighteenth year in females and nineteenth year in males.
The greater trochanter appears in the fourth year and fuses to the shaft in the eighteenth year in females and nineteenth year in males.
The lesser trochanter appears between the twelfth and fourteenth year and fuses to the shaft in the eighteenth year.
The lower extremity appears at the ninth month of intrauterine life and fuses to the shaft in the eighteenth year in females and twentieth year in males.

Pathology

Fracture of the neck of the femur is a common injury in people over 60 years of age, especially females. It may be pathological in origin, the upper extremity being weakened by metastatic deposits.

Pertrochanteric fracture occurs in the upper extremity between the two trochanters.

Subcapital fracture occurs just below the femoral head.

Legg-Calvé-Perthès' disease more commonly referred to as Perthès' disease, is osteochondritis of the capitular (head) epiphysis of the femur.

Osteogenic sarcoma is a malignant disease which most commonly occurs at the distal end of the femur. The disease most often presents in teenagers, the greatest occurrence being at 17 years.

Ewing's tumour occurs in the medullary cavity of a long bone. It is a childhood tumour. The primary site may arise in any part of a long bone, but the midshaft of the femur is the most common site.

Osteoclastoma or giant-cell tumour occurs most frequently in the 20 to 35 age group. It most often occurs at the lower end of femur and the upper end of the tibia.

THE PATELLA (Fig. 19)

Classification

The patella is a sesamoid bone.

Situation and articulations

The patella develops on the anterior aspect of the lower femur within the tendon of the quadriceps femoris muscle. It articulates with the patellar surface of the femur. When the knee is extended, the lower part of the patella lies 2.5 cm above the joint space of the knee.

Bone tissue

The patella is cancellous with a layer of compact bone.

Description

The patella is triangular in shape, the apex pointing inferiorly. It is flattened from front to back and therefore presents anterior and posterior surfaces, and superior, medial and lateral borders.

The *anterior surface* is convex with perforations for nutrient vessels and vertical grooves for the attachment of an extension of the quadriceps femoris tendon. Some fibres pass in the grooves to emerge as the superficial fibres of the patellar ligament.

The *posterior surface* is the articular surface. It is divided into two by a *median ridge,* which corresponds to the groove on the patellar surface of the femur. The medial articular surface of the patella is smaller than the lateral surface.

The *superior border* is thick and gives attachment to the part of the quadriceps femoris which is derived from the rectus femoris and vastus intermedius muscles.

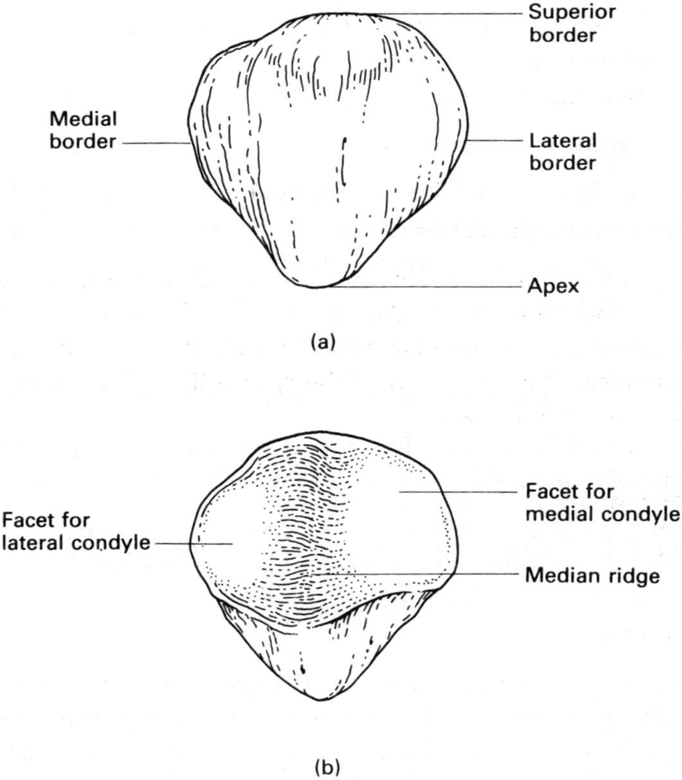

Fig. 19 Left patella — anterior (a) and posterior (b) aspects.

The *medial and lateral borders* are thinner than the superior border. They give attachment to the part of the quadriceps femoris which is derived from the vastus medialis and vastus lateralis muscles.

The *apex* points inferiorly and is roughened for the attachment of the patellar ligament.

Blood supply

The popliteal artery drains to the popliteal vein.

Nerve supply

The femoral nerve.

Ossification

The patella ossifies from several centres which appear in the third to sixth years; these centres quickly coalesce. Marginal centres appear later and fuse with the central mass.

Pathology

Fractures of the patella are commonly transverse in direction.

Bi-partite patella occurs when the upper outer quadrant ossifies separately and does not fuse with the rest of the patella.

Tri-partite patella occurs when, in addition to the upper outer quadrant, the outer lower aspect also ossifies separately and does not fuse.

THE FABELLA

The fabella is the name given to a sesamoid bone which occasionally develops in the gastrocnemius muscle behind the knee.

THE TIBIA (Figs. 20, 21 and 22)

Classification

The tibia is a long bone and therefore consists of an upper extremity, a shaft and a lower extremity.

Situation and articulations

The tibia is the medial bone of the lower leg. It is the second longest bone of the skeleton.
Superiorly it articulates with the condyles of the femur, forming part of the knee-joint, and with the fibula, forming the superior tibiofibular joint.
Inferiorly the tibia articulates with the talus, to form part of the ankle-joint, and with the fibula, to form the inferior tibiofibular joint.

Bone tissue

The shaft consists of compact bone surrounding a medullary cavity. The extremities are cancellous, surrounded by a thin layer of compact bone.

Description

The upper extremity

The upper extremity is expanded from side to side into two condyles, thus providing a large area for weight transference.

The *medial condyle* is the larger of the two condyles. It projects backwards, slightly overhanging the shaft. The articular surface is oval in shape and slightly concave to articulate with the medial condyle of the femur.

The *lateral condyle* also projects backwards, slightly overhanging the shaft. It bears on its postero-lateral surface a facet for articulation with the fibula. The articular area for the lateral condyle of the femur is circular in shape and slightly concave.

The *intercondylar area* is a roughened area on the superior surface of the tibia between the condyles. It is divided into three parts: the anterior intercondylar area, the intercondylar eminence and the posterior intercondylar area. It gives attachment to the medial and lateral menisci and to the cruciate ligaments of the knee-joint.

The *tibial tuberosity* is situated on the anterior border of the upper shaft. It is a triangular-shaped area which is easily palpable. It gives attachment to the patellar ligament.

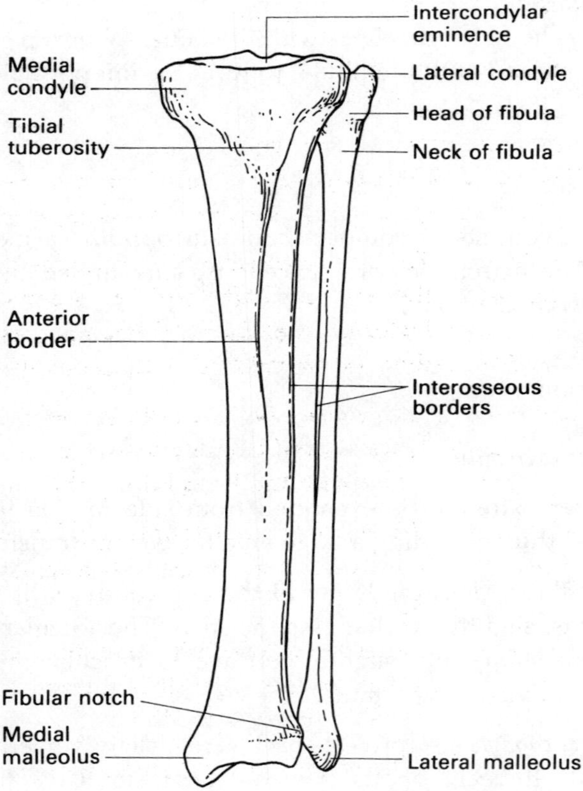

Fig. 20 Left tibia and fibula — anterior aspect.

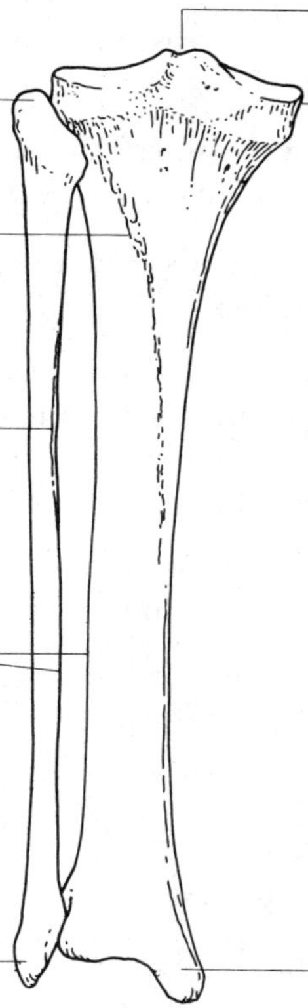

Fig. 21 Left tibia and fibula — posterior aspect.

The shaft

The shaft of the tibia is triangular in cross-section and presents medial, lateral and posterior surfaces and anterior, postero-medial and postero-lateral borders.

The *medial surface* is bounded by the anterior and postero-medial borders. It is palpable along nearly its entire length.

The *lateral surface* is bounded by the anterior and postero-lateral borders. The upper three-quarters is slightly concave from front to back and faces laterally. The lower quarter turns to face anteriorly.

The *posterior surface* is bounded by the postero-medial and postero-lateral borders. It is crossed by an oblique ridge called the *soleal line*.

The *anterior border* is very superficial and forms the shin. It extends from the tibial tuberosity to the medial malleolus.

The *postero-medial border* extends from the medial condyle to the medial malleolus of the tibia.

The *postero-lateral border* is the interosseus border. It gives attachment to the interosseus membrane between the tibia and the fibula. It extends from the fibular facet on the lateral condyle of the tibia to the anterior border of the fibular notch.

The *nutrient foramen* is usually located on the posterior surface of the tibia, inferior to the soleal line.

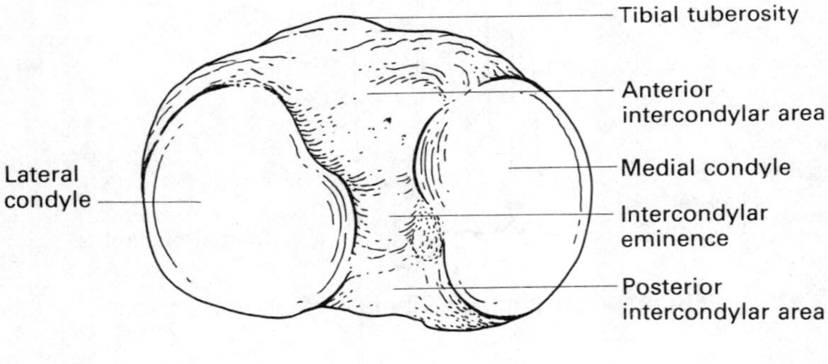

Fig. 22 Left tibia — superior aspect of the upper extremity.

The lower extremity

The lower extremity is expanded to present medial, lateral, posterior, anterior and inferior surfaces.

The *medial surface* is smooth and is continuous above with the medial surface of the shaft and below with the malleolus.

The *lateral surface* forms the triangular-shaped area termed the *fibular notch*. This area corresponds to an area on the fibula and forms the inferior tibiofibular joint.

The *posterior surface* is continuous above with the posterior surface of the shaft. It is crossed by a groove.

The *anterior surface* is smooth and is continuous above with the lateral surface of the tibial shaft.

The *inferior surface* is smooth for articulation with the body of the talus. It is concave from front to back and convex from side to side.

The *medial malleolus* is a pear-shaped process, the lateral surface of which articulates with the medial surface of the talus.

Blood supply

The posterior tibial artery drains to the posterior tibial vein.

Nerve supply

Tibial nerve.

Ossification

The shaft appears at the seventh week of intrauterine life.
The upper extremity appears at full term and fuses to the shaft in the sixteenth year in females and eighteenth year in males.
The lower extremity appears in the first year and fuses to the shaft in the fifteenth year in females and seventeenth year in males. The medial malleolus sometimes has its own centre of ossification.

Pathology

Osgood-Schlatter disease is osteochondritis of the tibial tuberosity.

Fractures have a tendency to be compound in type because the tibia is mainly superficial. They are usually in association with fractures of the fibula (see pathology of the fibula).

Fatigue fracture of the upper end of the tibia may occur due to prolonged walking.

THE FIBULA (Figs. 20 and 21)

Classification

The fibula is a long bone and therefore consists of an upper extremity, a shaft and a lower extremity.

Situation and articulations

The fibula is the lateral bone of the lower leg. It has no function in weight bearing and plays no part in the formation of the knee-joint, but is an important component of the ankle-joint. Superiorly it articulates with the tibia, to form the superior tibiofibular joint. Inferiorly it articulates with the tibia, to form the inferior tibiofibular joint, and with the talus, to form part of the ankle-joint.

Bone tissue

The shaft is compact bone surrounding a medullary cavity. The extremities are cancellous, surrounded by a thin layer of compact bone.

Description

The upper extremity

The head possesses a circular facet on its upper surface which articulates with the facet on the lateral condyle of the tibia. The apex of the head, sometimes called the *styloid process,* projects upwards from the postero-lateral part of the head.

The neck is a constriction separating the head from the shaft.

The shaft

The shaft possesses three surfaces and three borders, each of which is associated with muscles of the calf.

The *medial border* is the interosseus border which gives attachment to the interosseus membrane between the tibia and the fibula.

The *posterior surface* is divided into two at its upper part by a longitudinal ridge called the *median crest*. The lower part of the posterior surface turns to face medially and bears a facet for articulation with the fibular notch of the tibia.

The *nutrient foramen* is situated close to the median crest near to the mid-point of the shaft.

The lower extremity

The *lateral malleolus* projects further downwards and is more posterior than the medial malleolus of the tibia. Its medial surface bears a triangular-shaped facet for articulation with the talus. Behind this facet is a depression called the *malleolar fossa*.

Blood supply

The peroneal artery drains to the peroneal vein.

Nerve supply

Branches of the common peroneal nerve.

Ossification

The shaft appears at the eighth week of intrauterine life.
The upper extremity appears in the third year in females and fourth year in males and fuses with the shaft in the seventeenth year in females and nineteenth year in males.
The lower extremity appears in the first year and fuses to the

shaft in the fifteenth year in females and seventeenth year in males.

Pathology

Fractures. A displaced fracture of one of the bones of the lower leg is rare without a fracture or dislocation of the other bone, e.g. a fracture of the lower end of the tibia frequently causes a fracture of the neck of the fibula.

Pott's fracture is classified according to its severity. First degree is when the lateral malleolus only is fractured. Second degree is when there are fractures of both malleoli. Third degree is when, in addition to the fractures, there is a dislocation at the ankle-joint, due to a fracture of the posterior part of the medial malleolus.

Rickets is a childhood disease due usually to vitamin D and calcium deficiency. Although rickets may eventually affect all bones, one of its first effects is on the tibia and fibula, producing a bowed effect with characteristic knotting of the bone.

THE FOOT (Figs. 23 and 24)

The foot is composed of three groups of bones: the phalanges, metatarsals and tarsal bones.

The phalanges

The phalanges of the foot are similar in number and arrangement to those of the hand. The first or great toe has a distal and proximal phalanx. The other four toes have three: distal, middle and proximal phalanges.

Classification

The phalanges are long bones and therefore consist of a shaft and two extremities. The proximal extremity is known as the base and the distal extremity as the head.

Articulations

The bases of the proximal phalanges articulate with the corresponding metatarsals.

The heads of the proximal phalanges articulate with the bases of the middle phalanges (except for the first toe which, of course, has no middle phalanx).

The heads of the middle phalanges articulate with the bases of the distal phalanges.

Bone tissue

The shaft is compact bone surrounding a medullary cavity. The extremities are cancellous, surrounded by a thin layer of compact bone.

Description

The proximal phalanges

The shafts of the proximal phalanges are convex dorsally and concave on the plantar aspect. The bases are concave for articulation with the heads of the metatarsals. Each head presents a trochlear surface for articulation with the middle phalanx.

The middle phalanges

The middle phalanges are short and small.

The distal phalanges

The distal phalanges are small and flat. The bases have articular surfaces corresponding to those on the heads of the middle phalanges. The heads of the distal phalanges are expanded to support the pulp of the toe.

The metatarsals

The five metatarsal bones connect the tarsal bones to the phalanges. They are numbered one to five from the medial side.

Classification

The metatarsals are long bones and therefore consist of a shaft and two extremities. The proximal extremity is known as the base and the distal extremity as the head.

Articulations

The heads of the metatarsals articulate with the bases of the proximal phalanges of the corresponding toe.

The bases articulate with each other and with the tarsal bones as follows.

The first metatarsal articulates with the medial cuneiform and second metatarsal.
The second metatarsal articulates with the intermediate cuneiform, medial cuneiform, lateral cuneiform, first metatarsal and third metatarsal.
The third metatarsal articulates with the lateral cuneiform, second metatarsal and fourth metatarsal.
The fourth metatarsal articulates with the cuboid, lateral cuneiform, third metatarsal and fifth metatarsal.
The fifth metatarsal articulates with the cuboid and fourth metatarsal.

Bone tissue

The shaft is compact bone surrounding a medullary cavity. The extremities are cancellous, surrounded by a thin layer of compact bone.

Description

The first metatarsal is the shortest and thickest metatarsal; it bears two facets on the plantar surface of the head for articulation with two sesamoid bones. The second metatarsal is the longest of the metatarsals. The fifth metatarsal is characterized by a tuberosity, sometimes called the styloid process, on the lateral side of the base.

The tarsal bones

The tarsal bones consist of seven bones arranged in two rows. The proximal row consists of the talus and the calcaneum, the distal row consists of the medial, intermediate and lateral cuneiforms and the cuboid. In addition to these bones, between the two rows on the medial side, is the navicular.

Classification

The tarsal bones are short bones.

Articulations

The talus articulates with the inferior surface of the tibia, lateral malleolus, medial malleolus, navicular and calcaneum.
The calcaneum articulates with the talus and cuboid.
The navicular articulates with the medial cuneiform, intermediate cuneiform, lateral cuneiform, talus and occasionally with the cuboid.
The medial cuneiform articulates with the navicular, base of the first metatarsal, base of the second metatarsal and intermediate cuneiform. The intermediate cuneiform articulates with the base of the second metatarsal, navicular, medial cuneiform and lateral cuneiform.
The lateral cuneiform articulates with the base of the fourth metatarsal, base of the third metatarsal, cuboid, navicular, intermediate cuneiform and base of the second metatarsal.

The cuboid articulates with the lateral cuneiform, calcaneum, base of the fourth metatarsal, base of the fifth metatarsal and occasionally with the navicular.

Bone tissue

The tarsal bones are cancellous bone with a thin layer of compact bone.

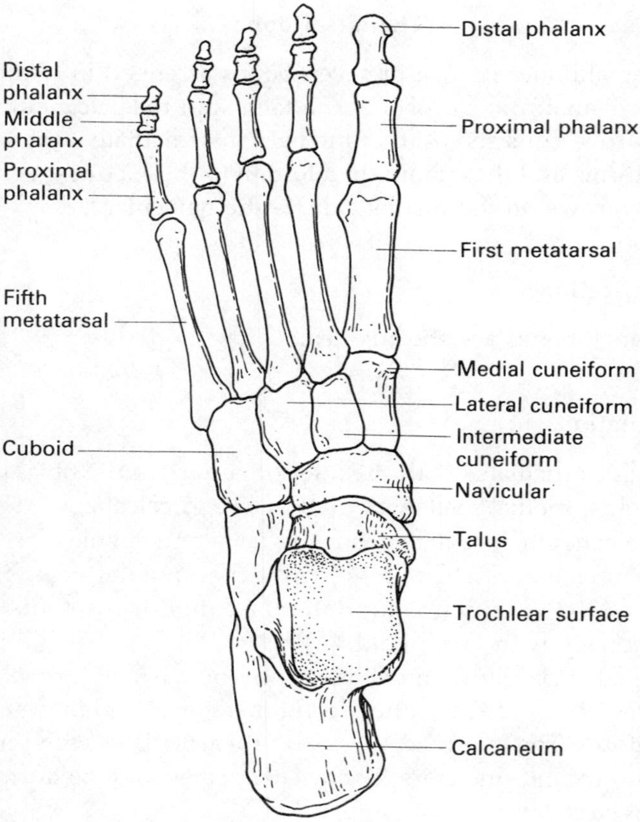

Fig. 23 Left foot — dorsal aspect.

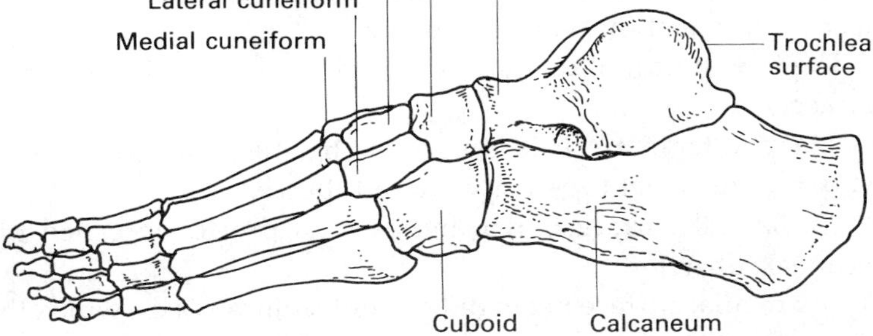

Fig. 24 Left foot — lateral aspect.

Description

The talus

The talus forms part of the ankle-joint and therefore connects the rest of the foot to the leg. Its head articulates distally with the navicular. The plantar surface of the head articulates with a shelf of bone on the calcaneum called the sustentaculum tali. The plantar surface also articulates with another facet of the calcaneum and with the navicular. The head is connected to the body of the talus by the neck. The body has a distinctive trochlear surface for articulation with the lower end of the tibia. The lateral surface articulates with the lateral malleolus and the medial surface with the medial malleolus. The posterior surface bears a roughened projection called the posterior process. The plantar surface has an oval facet for articulation with the calcaneum.

The calcaneum

The calcaneum is the largest of the tarsal bones. It forms the heel of the foot.

The dorsal surface has an anterior facet and a larger posterior facet for articulation with the talus. The dorsal surface also presents a middle articular facet for the talus.

The anterior surface is the smallest surface and presents a facet for articulation with the cuboid.

The lowest part of the posterior surface is the weight-bearing surface.

The plantar surface is rough for ligament attachments. It bears the calcaneal tuberosity and a tubercle.

The lateral surface is flat and bears a projection called the peroneal tubercle.

The medial surface bears the sustentaculum tali on which the talus sits.

The navicular

The navicular lies between the distal and proximal rows of the tarsal bones.

The distal surface is convex with three facets for articulation with the cuneiform bones.

The proximal surface is concave for articulation with the talus.

The medial surface bears a tuberosity.

The lateral surface is rough and irregular, sometimes presenting a facet for articulation with the cuboid.

The medial cuneiform

The distal surface of the medial cuneiform has a facet for articulation with the base of the first metatarsal.

The proximal surface articulates with the navicular.

The lateral surface bears two facets, one for the intermediate cuneiform and one for the base of the second metatarsal.

The intermediate cuneiform

The distal surface of the intermediate cuneiform articulates with the base of the second metatarsal.

The proximal surface has a facet for articulation with the navicular.

The medial surface articulates with the medial cuneiform.

The lateral surface has a facet for articulation with the lateral cuneiform.

The lateral cuneiform

The distal surface of the lateral cuneiform articulates with the base of the third metatarsal.

The proximal surface articulates with the navicular.

The medial surface has two facets, one articulating with the intermediate cuneiform, the other with the base of the second metatarsal.

The lateral surface has two facets, one for the cuboid and one for the base of the fourth metatarsal.

The cuboid

The cuboid is the lateral bone of the distal row.

The medial surface articulates with the lateral cuneiform and occasionally with the navicular.

The distal surface articulates with the bases of the fourth and fifth metatarsals.

The proximal surface articulates with the distal surface of the calcaneum.

Essential aspects of the foot

Blood supply

The foot is supplied by branches of the peroneal, anterior tibial and posterior tibial arteries draining to the veins of the same name.

Nerve supply

Branches of the tibial, deep peroneal (anterior tibial) and superficial peroneal nerves.

Ossification

The *phalanges* ossify from two centres, one each for the shaft and the base. The shafts of the distal phalanges appear at the ninth to twelfth week of intrauterine life.
The shafts of the middle phalanges appear after the fifteenth week of intrauterine life.
The shafts of the proximal phalanges appear at the eleventh to fifteenth week of intrauterine life.
The epiphyses of the phalanges appear between the second and eighth year and unite with the shaft at approximately the eighteenth year.

The *metatarsals* ossify from two centres. The first metatarsal has centres for the shaft and base, the other metatarsals having centres for the shaft and head.
The shafts appear at the ninth to tenth week of intrauterine life.
The epiphyses appear between the third and fourth year and unite with the shaft between the seventeenth and twentieth years.

The *tarsals* ossify from a single centre, except for the calcaneum.
The calcaneum appears at the third month of intrauterine life.
The epiphysis appears in the sixth year in females and eighth year in males, uniting in the fourteenth year in females and sixteenth year in males.
The talus appears at the sixth month of intrauterine life.
The cuboid appears at birth.
The lateral cuneiform appears in the first year of life.
The medial cuneiform appears in the second year.
The intermediate cuneiform and the navicular appear in the third year.

Pathology

Pes planus is a deformity of the foot whereby the bony relationship is changed and the longitudinal arch lowers.

Os trigonum is the name given to the variant in ossification when the posterior process of the talus ossifies separately and does not unite with the rest of the talus.

March fracture is a type of stress fracture (due to prolonged walking) occuring in one or more metatarsals.

Koehler's disease is juvenile osteochondritis of the navicular.

Gout is due to an excessive amount of uric acid which frequently collects as urate crystals around the first metatarso-phalangeal joint.

SELF–TEST

1 State the articulations of the femur.
2 Describe the shape of the head of the femur.
3 The fovea gives attachment to which ligament?
4 State the position of the adductor tubercle.
5 What is Legg-Calvé-Perthès' disease?
6 The patella develops in the tendon of which muscle?
7 Describe the shape of the patella.
8 Name the ridge which divides the posterior surface of the patella.
9 What is a fabella?
10 Which tibial condyle bears a facet for articulation with the fibula?
11 What is Osgood-Schlatter disease?
12 State the articulations of the fibula.
13 What is the name of the crest which divides the posterior surface of the fibula?
14 Which is the longest metatarsal?
15 List the tarsal bones.
16 What is pes planus?

Check your answers against those given at the back of the book.

CHAPTER 5
THE BONES OF THE PELVIC GIRDLE

The pelvis is a bony ring composed of two hip bones, forming the anterior and lateral walls, and the sacrum and coccyx, which together form the posterior wall. Descriptions of the sacrum and coccyx are given in Chapter 6. Below is a description of the hip bone.

THE HIP BONE (Fig. 25)

Classification

The hip bone is classified as a flat bone.

Situation and articulations

The hip bones form the anterior and lateral walls of the pelvis
The ilium of the hip bone articulates with the sacrum, forming the sacroiliac joint.
The acetabulum of the hip bone articulates with the head of the femur, forming the hip-joint.
In the midline is the articulation between the pubis of each hip bone. This is the symphysis pubis.

Bone tissue

The hip bone consists of two layers of compact bone with a layer of cancellous between.

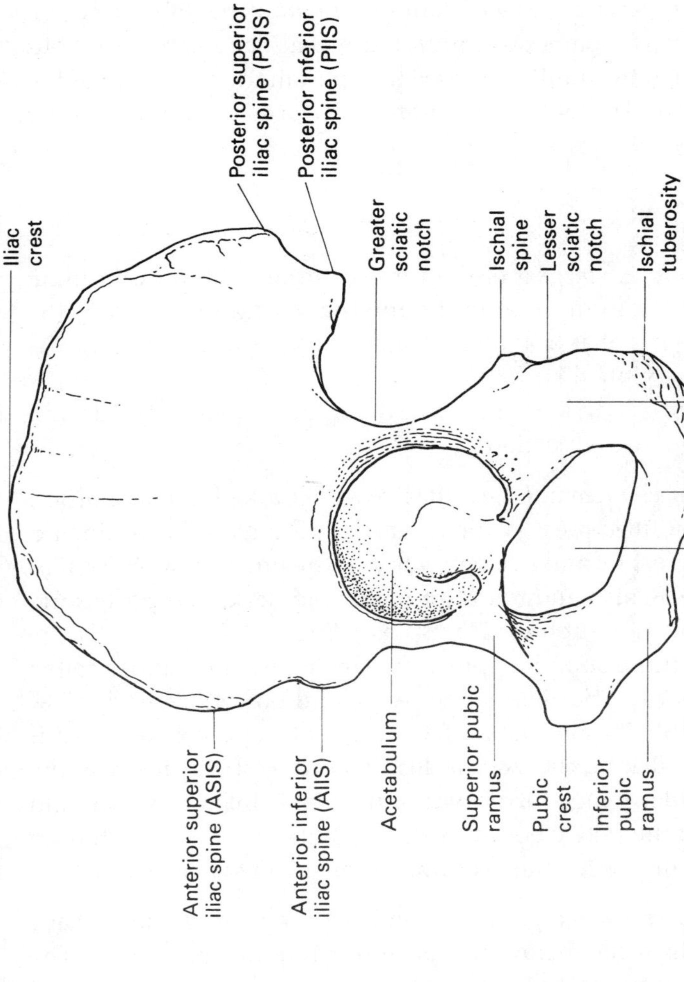

Fig. 25 Left hip bone — external aspect.

Description

The hip bone is a large, irregularly shaped flat bone. It is dominated by two features: a hemispherical depression called the acetabulum and an oval hole in the bone called the obturator foramen.

The hip bone is formed from three parts: the ilium, ischium and pubis. The parts are connected by cartilage in children but are united in the adult. All three take part in the formation of the acetabulum. The obturator foramen is formed by the ischium and pubis.

The ilium

The ilium is the largest of the three component bones, forming two-thirds of the hip bone. Its internal surface is smooth; the external surface is roughened for muscle attachments and is termed the gluteal surface.

The ilium is divided into two: the upper expanded blade and the lower narrow portion.

The *upper expanded blade* has a well-marked upper border, termed the iliac crest, which is an important bony landmark. The iliac crest terminates anteriorly in the anterior superior iliac spine (ASIS) also an important bony landmark, and posteriorly in the posterior superior iliac spine (PSIS).

Below these superior spines are smaller inferior spines called the anterior inferior iliac spine (AIIS) and posterior inferior iliac spine (PIIS). Its internal surface is smooth and concave and is called the iliac fossa. At the lower border of the fossa is the pelvic border which forms part of the pelvic inlet. Posterior and inferior to the pelvic border is the auricular surface, which is an articular surface for the sacrum, forming the sacroiliac joint.

The *lower narrow portion* is narrowed by the greater sciatic notch, which lies below the posterior inferior iliac spine. The roof and upper part of the acetabulum is formed by this part of the ilium.

The ischium

The ischium forms the inferior and posterior part of the hip bone. It consists of a body, ramus, spine and tuberosity.

The *body* forms the lower posterior part of the acetabulum and supports the weight when sitting down.

The *ramus* arises from the body and extends superiorly to unite with the inferior pubic ramus. The ischial ramus forms the lower border of the obturator foramen.

The *ischial spine* arises from the body. It forms the lower margin of the greater sciatic notch and the upper margin of the lesser sciatic notch.
The *ischial tuberosity* marks the inferior portion of the body.

The pubis

The pubis is the smallest of the three parts of the hip bone; it forms the inferior and anterior part. It consists of a body and two rami.

The *body* is in close proximity to the urinary bladder. It is a flat portion of bone, the superior border of which is easily palpable as the pubic crest. The symphysis pubis is formed by the articulation of the pubic bodies on each side.

The *superior and inferior pubic rami* arise from the body. The superior pubic ramus extends superiorly and laterally to form part of the acetabulum. The inferior pubic ramus extends inferiorly and posteriorly to join with the ischial ramus.

The acetabulum (Fig. 26)

The acetabulum is a hemispherical depression situated on the external surface of the hip bone. The three parts of the hip bone unite here in the shape of a Y. The ilium forms the superior two-fifths of the articular part of the acetabulum. The ischium forms the inferoposterior two-fifths and the pubis forms the

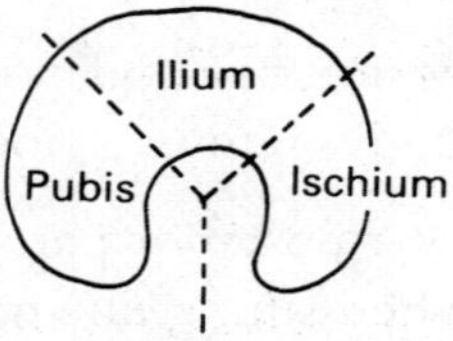

Fig. 26 Left acetabulum.

inferoanterior one-fifth of the acetabulum The bony rim is deficient inferiorly at the acetabular notch.

The rim is deepened by fibrocartilage.

The obturator foramen (Fig. 27)

The obturator foramen is formed by the superior and inferior pubic rami, ischial ramus and body of the ischium.

The foramen is enclosed by a membrane and is pierced by nerves and blood vessels of the buttocks and legs.

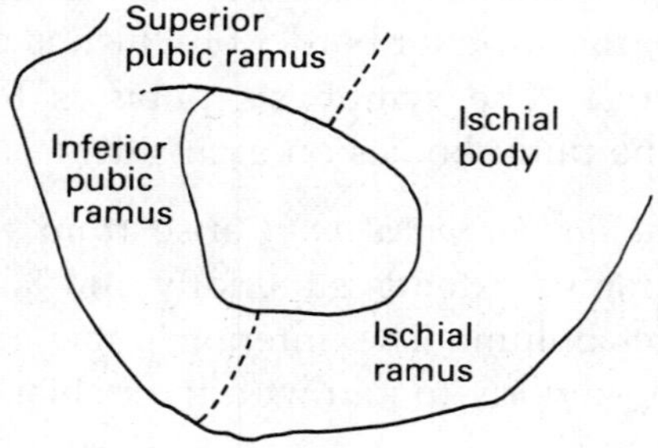

Fig. 27 Left obturator foramen.

Blood supply

Branches of the internal and external iliac arteries drain to the veins of the same name.

Nerve supply

Branches from the lumbar, sacral and coccygeal plexi.

Ossification

The hip bone ossifies from eight centres: three primary and five secondary. The primary centres are the ilium (appears at eight to nine weeks) ischium (appears in the third month of intrauterine life) and the pubis (appears at four to five months). By the thirteenth to fourteenth year of life, growth in these centres has extended to the bottom of the acetabulum. The centres are then separated from each other by a Y-shaped cartilage. This cartilage (a secondary centre) then ossifies, completing the acetabulum. The other secondary centres of ossification are the iliac crest, anterior inferior spinous process, ischial tuberosity and symphysis pubis. These appear at puberty, to unite between the twentieth and twenty-fifth years.

Pathology

See end of this chapter.

THE PELVIS

Functions

1 Protection of the lower abdominal and pelvic organs, i.e. bladder, rectum, female organs of reproduction and parts of the small and large bowel.

2 Weight transference; this is achieved by the bone structure and the ligaments of the pelvis.

(a) Weight transference on standing. Weight is transferred via the vertebral column to the sacrum and thus to the right and left sacroiliac joints. Weight is then transferred along the pelvic border of the ilium to the acetabulum and head of the femur.

(b) Weight transference on sitting. The same route of

weight transference applies as above but from the pelvic border of the ilium weight is transferred to the bodies of the ischium.

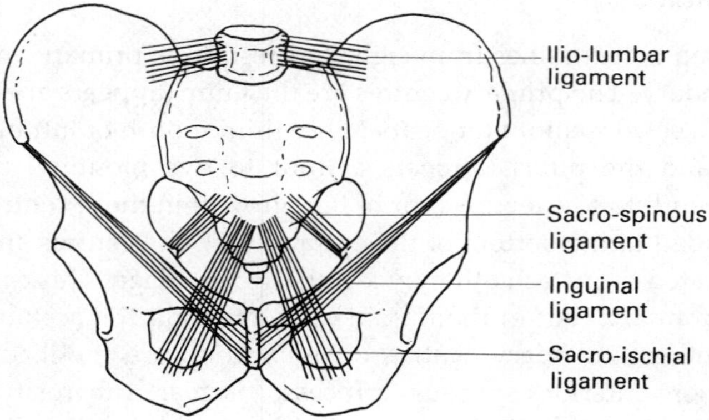

Fig. 28 Major ligaments of the pelvis.

The ligaments of the pelvis (Fig. 28)

The four most important ligaments of the pelvis are the:
1 ilio-lumbar ligament (the fifth lumbar vertebra to the ilium);
2 inguinal ligament (the anterior superior iliac spine to the pubic tubercle);
3 sacro-spinous ligament (the sacrum to the ischial tuberosity); and
4 sacro-ischial ligament (the sacrum to the ischium).

True and false pelves

The pelvis is divided into the false or greater pelvis and the true or lesser pelvis by the pelvic inlet.

The pelvic inlet (Fig. 29)

The pelvic inlet is formed by the promontory of the sacrum, pelvic border of ilium and upper border of the pubis. The false

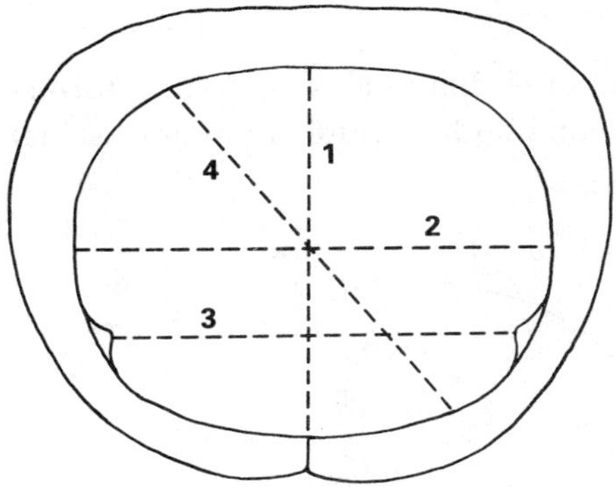

Fig. 29 Dimensions of the pelvic inlet as demonstrated on a pelvic inlet radiograph. 1, true conjugate; 2, transverse; 3, interspinous; 4, oblique.

pelvis is continuous with the true pelvis through the pelvic inlet. The size of the pelvic inlet is of obstetric importance and by radiographic examination — 'pelvimetry' — the following measurements may be made:

1 true conjugate — the distance from the sacral promontory to the upper border of the symphysis pubis;

2 transverse — the maximum distance between two similar points;

3 interspinous — the distance between ischial spines, and;

4 oblique — the distance from the sacroiliac joint to the opposite ilio-pubic eminence.

The true pelvis

The true pelvis or pelvic cavity is bounded above by the pelvic inlet. It is funnel shaped, the posterior bony wall being longer, and contains the bladder, rectum, sigmoid colon and female organs of reproduction. It is bounded below by the outlet.

The pelvic outlet

The pelvic outlet is diamond shaped and formed by the tip of the coccyx, ischial bodies, pubic rami and ischial rami.

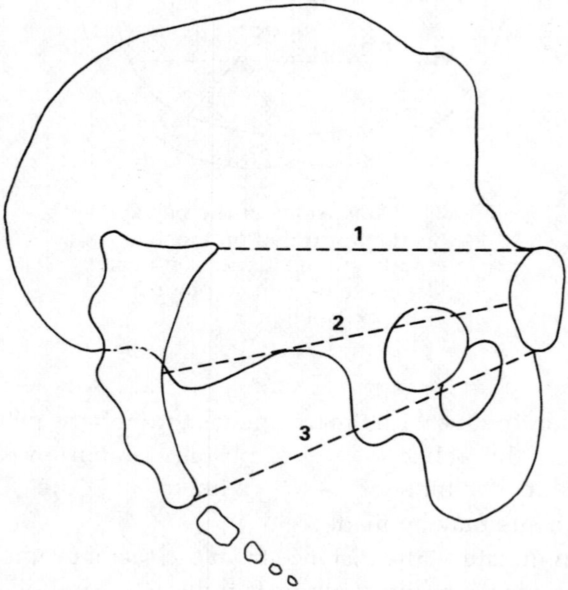

Fig. 30 Planes of the female pelvis as demonstrated on a lateral pelvimetry radiograph.

Planes of the true pelvis (Fig. 30)

Pelvimetry may be undertaken to ascertain the dimensions of the true pelvis. On a lateral pelvimetry radiograph the following planes may be measured:

1 true conjugate — the distance from the sacral promontory to the upper symphysis pubis;

2 midplane — the distance from the middle of the third sacral segment to the mid-point of the symphysis pubis; and

3 outlet — the distance from the last moveable joint to the lower part of the symphysis pubis. (N.B. the last moveable joint is usually the sacrococcygeal joint but sometimes the coccyx is fused to the sacrum and the last moveable joint may be between the segments of the coccyx.)

Comparison of male and female pelves

The differences between the typical male and typical female pelvis are associated with the obstetric requirements of the female pelvis. The main differences are summarized in Table 1.

Table 1 The differences between the typical male and female pelves.

Typical male pelvis	Typical female pelvis
Bigger overall dimensions	Smaller overall dimensions
Well-ridged muscle attachments	Less well-ridged muscle attachments
Sub-pubic arch narrow	Sub-pubic arch wide
Ischial spines close together	Ischial spines wider apart
Inlet small and triangular	Inlet large and round
Pelvic cavity long and narrow	Pelvic cavity short with straight walls which are wide apart
Sacrum curved	Sacrum less curved

Pathology

Congenital dislocation of the hip (CDH) is a congenital deformity where there is dislocation or subluxation of the hip-joint due to defective development of the acetabulum.

Malgaigne's fracture is a vertical fracture of the posterior pelvic wall associated with a dislocation of the sacroiliac joint of the same side.

Osteomalacia, sometimes called adult rickets, is a condition which often first presents in the pelvis.

Paget's disease is an idiopathic, skeletal disease causing porotic changes in the early stages but an increase in thickness and density of bone in the more advanced stage.

An *asymmetrical pelvis* may be due to a variety of causes, e.g. scoliosis, CDH. In females it may cause obstetric difficulties.

Fractures. Because the pelvis is a bony ring, severe trauma frequently causes fractures on both sides or a fracture on one side associated with a dislocation of the sacroiliac joint of the opposite side or dislocation of the symphysis pubis.

NB When dealing with patients with pelvic injuries one must remember the danger of soft-tissue damage by the fracture fragments on the closely related organs, e.g. the bladder, urethra and rectum.

SELF–TEST

1 Classify the hip bone.
2 Name the three parts of the hip bone.
3 Name the parts of the hip bone forming the obturator foramen.
4 What structure supports the body weight when sitting?
5 List the functions of the pelvis.
6 Which structures form the pelvic inlet?
7 Where is the true conjugate?
8 Describe the shape of a typical female pelvic inlet.
9 What does the abbreviation CDH mean?
10 What structures are at risk in pelvic fractures?

Check your answers against those given at the back of the book.

CHAPTER 6
THE VERTEBRAL COLUMN

The vertebral column consists of 26 irregular bones articulated together. The parts of the column are as follows:

Cervical vertebrae	7
Thoracic vertebrae	12
Lumbar vertebrae	5
Sacrum	1
Coccyx	1

Functions of the vertebral column

1 To protect the spinal cord.
2 To provide support for the head and trunk and allow for a certain flexibility of movement.
3 To transfer weight.
4 To give attachment to muscles.
5 To provide articulation for the ribs.

Curvatures of the vertebral column

The spine consists of four antero-posterior curvatures: two primary curves and two secondary curves.

The primary curves are so called because they are present at birth. They are the curves of the thoracic spine and the sacrum and coccyx and are convex posteriorly.

The secondary curves develop after birth. The cervical curvature develops in the first year of life as the baby begins to hold the head upright. The lumbar curvature develops in the second year of life as the child begins to hold the body upright.

The secondary curves are convex anteriorly.

The curves aid in the transmission of stress along the vertebral column. It is interesting to note that the secondary curves tend to disappear in old age, so that the body gradually reverts to its original shape of the spine being convex posteriorly.

The normal vertebral column has no lateral curvatures.

Articulations of the spine

The vertebral column has two sets of joints. These are the small synovial joints between adjacent articulating processes and fibrocartilaginous joints between the vertebral bodies and intervertebral discs.

Intervertebral discs

Discs are present between the bodies of each vertebra, except between the first and second cervical vertebrae. They form one-quarter of the total length of the vertebral column. Their function is to act as shock absorbers and thus to aid in weight transference. They are thickest in the lumbar region and thinnest in the thoracic region, where there is less movement compared to other parts of the spine.

The shape of each intervertebral disc corresponds to that of the vertebral body in contact with it. A thin, external layer of hyaline cartilage fixes the intervertebral disc to the adjacent vertebral body. Each consists of an outer ring of fibrous tissue, including a small amount of fibrocartilage; this is called the annulus fibrosis. The middle of the disc is a soft, gelatinous matrix called the nucleus pulposus. Intervertebral discs are avascular structures.

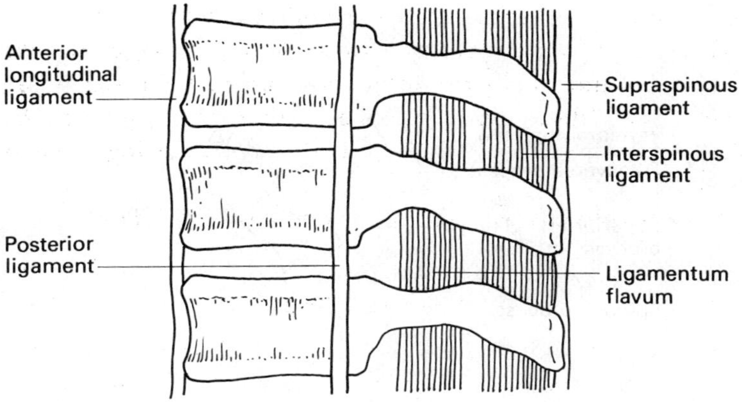

Fig. 31 Section through the vertebral column showing the ligaments.

Spinal ligaments (Fig. 31)

To add strength to the vertebral column there are the following ligaments.

The *anterior longitudinal ligament* extends from the first cervical vertebra to the sacrum in front of the anterior vertebral bodies and intervertebral discs.

The *posterior longitudinal ligament* extends from the first cervical vertebra to the sacrum behind the posterior vertebral bodies and intervertebral discs.

The *supraspinous ligament* extends from the seventh cervical vertebra to the sacrum connecting the tips of the spinous processes.

The *ligamentum nuchae* (not shown) extends from the external occipital protuberence to the seventh cervical vertebra connecting the tips of the spinous processes.

The *ligamentum flavum* extends between the laminae of each adjacent vertebra.

The *interspinous ligament* extends between the spinous processes of each adjacent vertebra.

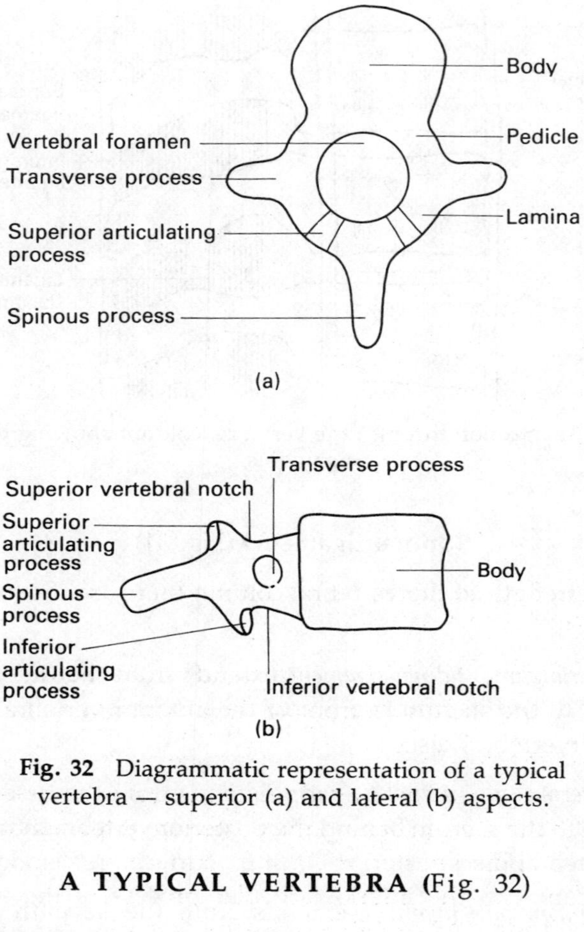

Fig. 32 Diagrammatic representation of a typical vertebra — superior (a) and lateral (b) aspects.

A TYPICAL VERTEBRA (Fig. 32)

Classification

The vertebrae are classified as being irregular bones.

Articulations

Each vertebra articulates with the vertebra above and below via the articular processes. The bodies are separated by intervertebral discs.

Bone tissue

Each vertebra is cancellous with a layer of compact bone.

Description

The *body* is the cylindrical, anterior part of the vertebra. It is convex anteriorly and concave posteriorly. The superior and inferior surfaces of the body are flat. These two surfaces are covered by hyaline cartilage.

The *right and left pedicles* project posteriorly from the body. They are short and round in cross-section.

The *right and left laminae* arise from the pedicles. They are directed posteriorly and medially to fuse in the midline.

The *transverse processes* project laterally, one on each side from the area where the pedicles fuse with the laminae. Their function is muscle attachment.

The *spinous process* is a single, midline structure arising from the point of fusion of the right and left laminae. It projects posteriorly and its function is muscle attachment.

The *articular processes* are four in number: a pair of superior articular processes and a pair of inferior articular processes. The superior articular processes are directed superiorly and posteriorly. The posterior facing surface is smooth for articulation with the inferior articular process of the vertebra above. The inferior articular processes are directed inferiorly and anteriorly. The anterior facing surface is smooth for articulation with the superior articular process of the vertebra below.

The *superior and inferior vertebral notches* are situated on the superior and inferior aspects of the pedicle and/or lamina. On articulation, the notches of adjacent vertebrae form the intervertebral foramina through which the spinal nerves leave the neural canal.

The *vertebral foramen* is formed by the posterior surface of the body, pedicles and laminae. The vertebral foramen transmits the spinal cord and its coverings. Articulated together, the channel formed by the spine is called the *neural canal*.

Blood supply

Blood supply is via branches derived from the vertebral and inferior thyroid arteries in the neck, from the intercostal arteries in the thorax and from the lumbar and lateral sacral arteries in the abdomen and pelvic regions.

Venous drainage is from a complicated network of veins surrounding the vertebrae and is ultimately to the vertebral veins in the neck, intercostal veins in the thorax and lumbar and sacral veins in the abdomen and pelvis.

Nerve supply

Nerve supply is from the posterior division of the spinal nerves as they emerge from the intervertebral foramina.

Ossification

Each vertebra ossifies from four primary centres: one for each lamina and two for the body. The laminae appear in the sixth week of intrauterine life; the body appears in the eighth week of intrauterine life. The three secondary centres appear in the sixteenth year, to unite by the twenty-fifth year. These centres are for the tip of each transverse process and the tip of the spinous process. *Note*: This is a simplification of the ossification of vertebrae; a full description may be found in *Gray's Anatomy*, (35th edn. Longman Group Ltd., Edinburgh, Scotland).

Pathology

See end of this chapter.

The common features of the vertebrae have been described: the discussion which follows concentrates only on the characteristic features which identify the vertebrae.

THE CERVICAL VERTEBRAE

There are seven cervical vertebrae, which are the smallest of the vertebrae. The first, second and seventh are considered to be atypical. The third, fourth, fifth and sixth are typical and can be described together.

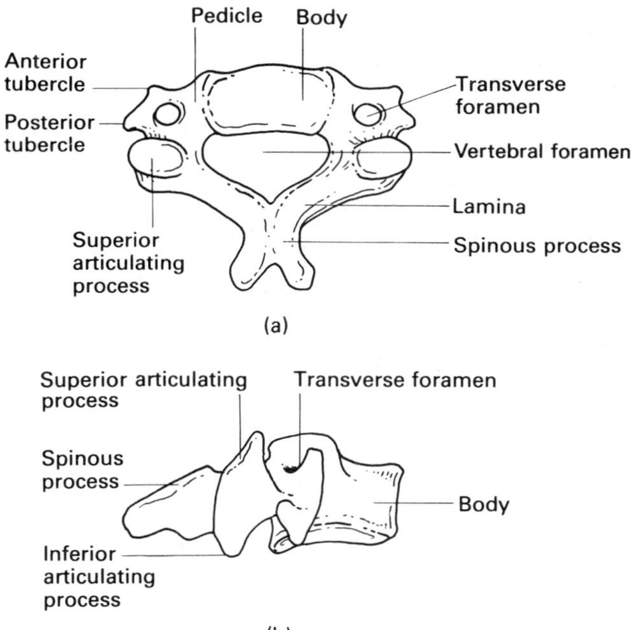

Fig. 33 A typical cervical vertebra — superior (a) and lateral oblique (b) aspects.

Typical (Fig. 33)

The *body* is small and oval. The inferior surface forms a prominent lip.

The *vertebral foramen* is relatively large compared to the body and is triangular in shape.

The *pedicles* are short and thick and project laterally and posteriorly.

The *transverse processes* are formed by an anterior and a posterior root which terminate in an anterior and a posterior tubercle enclosing a foramen called the transverse foramen. This transmits the vertebral artery.

The *spinous process* is flattened supero-inferiorly and has a bifid tip.

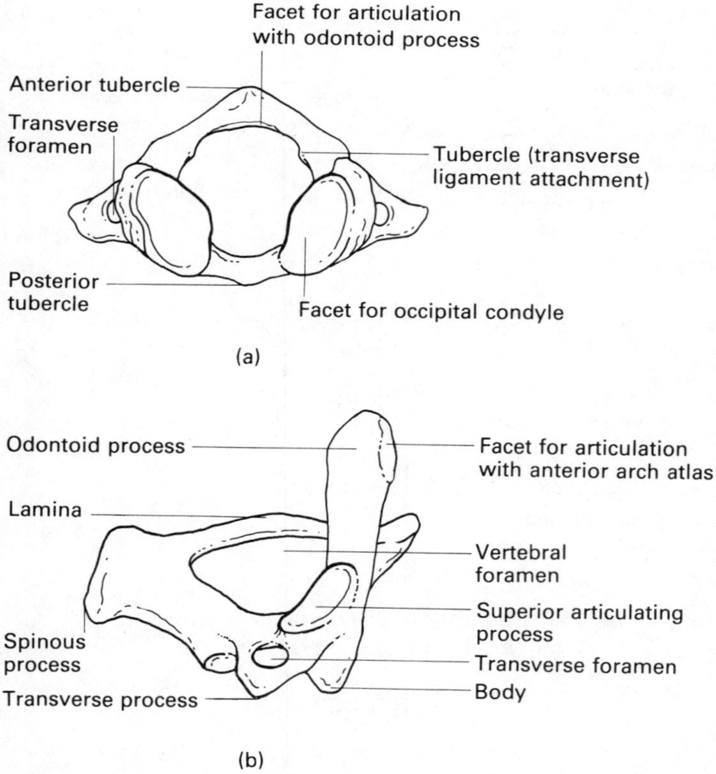

Fig. 34 Atlas — superior (a) and Axis — oblique lateral (b) aspects.

Atypical (Fig. 34)

The *first cervical vertebra* or *atlas* has no body or spinous process. It consists of an anterior and a posterior arch. The posterior surface of the anterior arch bears a facet for articulation with the odontoid process of the second cervical vertebra. The anterior surface of the anterior arch bears a small projection called the anterior tubercle. There is also a posterior tubercle projecting from the posterior surface of the posterior arch.

Separating the arches on either side are the lateral masses. On the superior aspect of each lateral mass is a large, kidney-shaped facet for articulation with the occipital condyle, forming the atlanto-occipital joint.

On the medial aspect of each lateral mass is a tubercle to which is attached the transverse ligament. This ligament helps to hold the odontoid process of the second cervical vertebra in place.

The *second cervical vertebra* or *axis* has a peg-like process on the superior aspect of the body called the odontoid process. The process has a facet on the anterior surface for articulation with the anterior arch of the first cervical vertebra and postero-inferiorly it is grooved by the transverse ligament of the atlas.

The *seventh cervical vertebra* has a spinous process which is long and not bifid. It is easily palpable and usually visible through the muscle and skin of the neck. The transverse foramina are small and do not transmit the vertebral arteries.

THE THORACIC VERTEBRAE

There are twelve thoracic vertebrae. The first, ninth, tenth, eleventh and twelfth are considered to be atypical. The second to eighth inclusive are typical and can be described together.

Typical (Fig. 35)

The *body* is heart shaped, with costal demi-facets on its superior and inferior sides. The superior demi-facet articulates with the

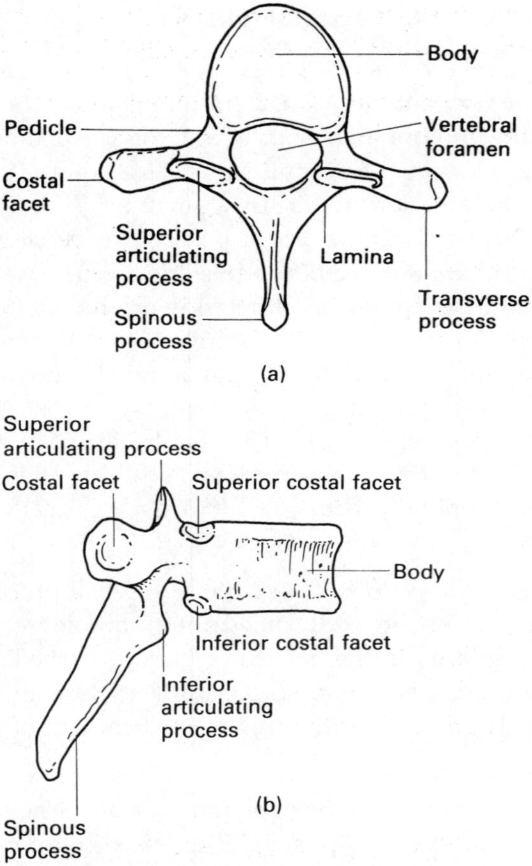

Fig. 35 A typical thoracic vertebra — superior (a) and lateral (b) aspects.

lower part of the head of the rib of the same number as the vertebra. The inferior demi-facet articulates with the upper part of the head of the rib whose number would be one greater than this vertebra.

The *vertebral foramen* is relatively small and is circular.

The *pedicles* are short, thick and horizontal in position.

The *transverse processes* are long, thick and directed posteriorly and laterally. At the free end is a costal facet for articulation with the tubercle of the rib of the same number as the vertebra.

The *spinous process* is long, slender and is directed downwards to overlap the vertebra below.

Atypical

The *first thoracic vertebra* has a full facet on the upper body for articulation with the head of the first rib, and a demi-facet below for the upper part of the head of the second rib.

The *ninth thoracic vertebra* articulates only with the ninth rib. It has no inferior demi-facet on the body.

The *tenth thoracic vertebra* has one full facet on the upper body for the head of the tenth rib. Sometimes it has no facets on the transverse processes.

The *eleventh thoracic vertebra* has one full facet on the body for articulation with the eleventh rib. It has no facet on the transverse processes.

The *twelfth thoracic vertebra* has one full facet on the body for articulation with the twelfth rib. It has no facet on the transverse processes.

THE LUMBAR VERTEBRAE

There are five lumbar vertebrae. They are the largest and strongest of the moveable vertebrae. The fifth is atypical but the first to fourth inclusive are typical and can be described together.

Typical (Fig. 36)

The *body* is large and kidney shaped.

The *vertebral foramen* is triangular and is larger than those of the other vertebrae.

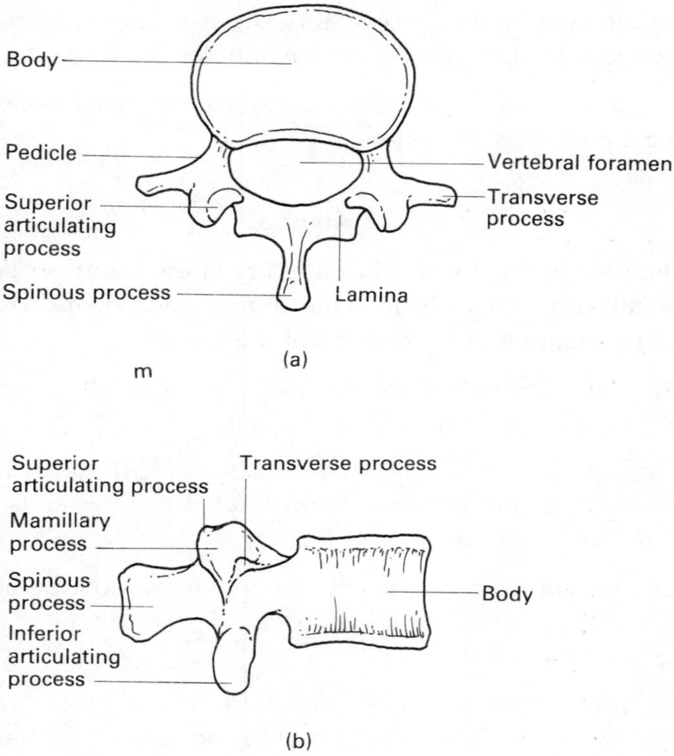

Fig. 36 A typical lumbar vertebra — superior (a) and lateral (b) aspects.

The *pedicles* are short, narrow and horizontal in position.

The *transverse processes* are relatively thin and elongated. At the root of each transverse process is a small tubercle called the accessory process.

The *spinous process* is short, quadrilateral and almost horizontal. Because the laminae are directed downwards as well as medially, it is at a lower level than the body.

The *inferior articular facets* face anteriorly and laterally and thus, by articulation with the *superior articular facets*, lateral movement of the vertebrae relative to each other is prevented. The superior articular processes bear a tubercle on the posterior surface called the mamillary process.

Atypical

The *fifth lumbar vertebra* has a body which is much deeper anteriorly than posteriorly. This accounts for the curvature at the junction of the fifth lumbar vertebra and the first sacral segment.

THE SACRUM (Figs. 37, 38 and 39)

The sacrum consists of five vertebrae fused together. Fusion occurs at approximately 14 years. It is triangular in shape with the base above and apex below.

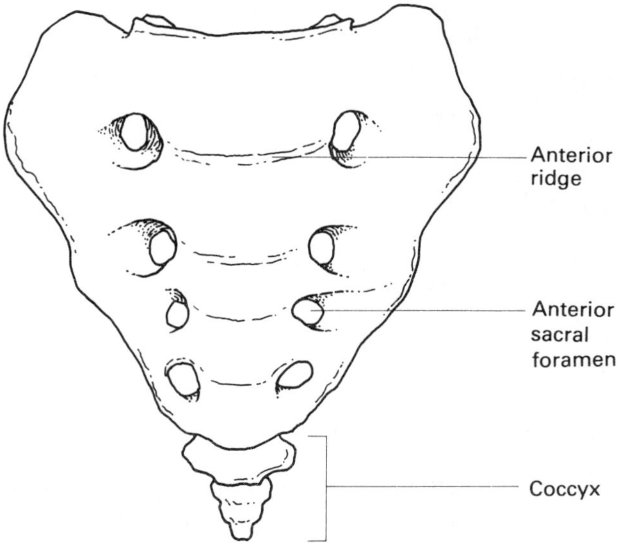

Fig. 37 Sacrum and coccyx — anterior aspect.

The anterior surface

The anterior surface is concave and smooth to support the pelvic organs. Four ridges cross the surface anteriorly. Lateral to the ridges are four pairs of anterior foramina which transmit the sacral nerves. They communicate with a central sacral canal. These foramina represent the intervertebral foramina of more conventional vertebrae. Lateral to them are the lateral masses. The lateral masses of the upper three segments unite to form the ala of the sacrum.

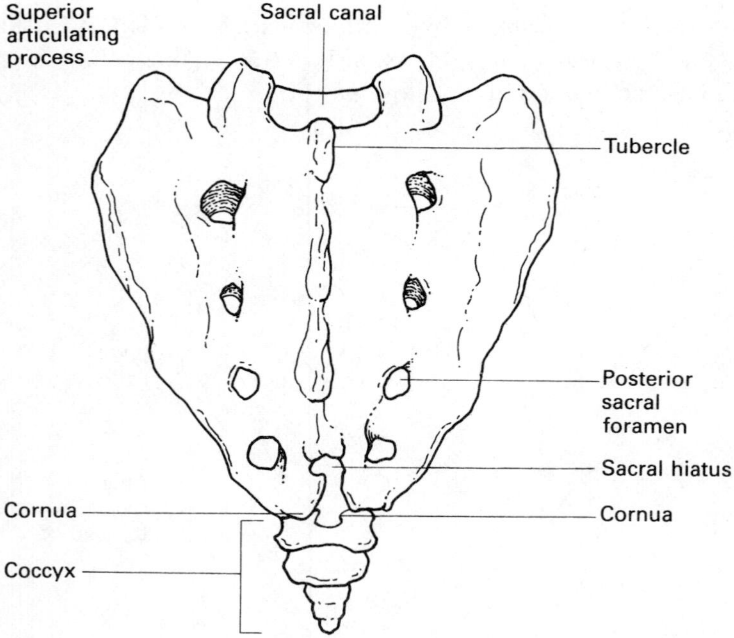

Fig. 38 Sacrum and coccyx — posterior aspect.

The posterior surface

The posterior surface is convex and roughened for muscle attachments. The spines of the vertebrae are represented by tubercles, which are joined by a ridge called the median crest.

Below the crest is a deficiency called the sacral hiatus. Lateral to the tubercles are the posterior sacral foramina which communicate with the sacral canal.

The first sacral segment presents a pair of superior articular processes which articulate with the inferior articular processes of the fifth lumbar vertebra.

The fifth sacral segment presents articular processes called cornua which project down on either side of the sacral hiatus.

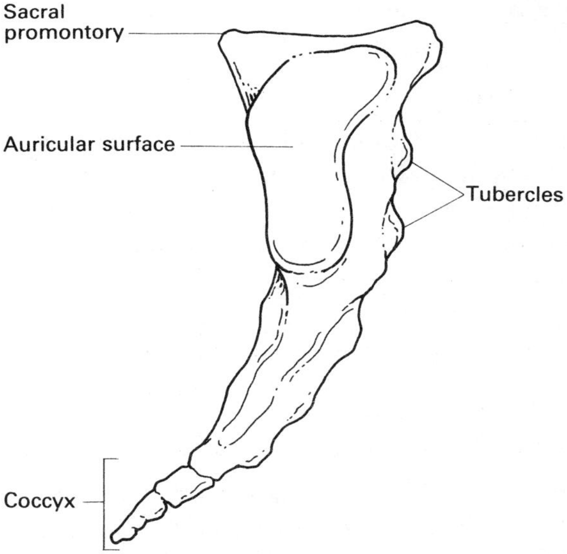

Fig. 39 Sacrum and coccyx — lateral aspect.

The base

The base faces superiorly and anteriorly. The body of the first sacral segment articulates with the body of the fifth lumbar vertebra. The anterior border of the body of the first sacral segment forms the sacral promontory. Behind the body is the triangular-shaped opening of the sacral canal.

The lateral surface

The lateral surface is wider above than below. The upper three segments form the auricular articular surface to articulate with the ilium of the hip bone, forming the sacroiliac joint. Behind the auricular surface is a roughened area for attachment of the sacroiliac ligaments.

The apex

The apex bears an oval facet for articulation with the coccyx.

THE COCCYX (Figs. 37, 38, and 39)

The coccyx consists of four fused segments, although occasionally there may be only three segments or sometimes as many as five. It is triangular with the base above and apex below. The base forms cornua which articulate with the cornua of the sacrum.

PATHOLOGY OF THE VERTEBRAL COLUMN

A *cervical rib* is a supernumerary rib which arises from the seventh cervical vertebra.

Ankylosing spondylitis is sometimes called bamboo spine. It is a condition whereby the spine fuses together, ultimately forming an inflexible column which resembles a bamboo pole. It usually commences in the sacroiliac joints.

Spina bifida is a developmental abnormality whereby the laminae do not fuse posteriorly. If symptomless, the condition is called spina bifida occulta.

Kyphosis is an exaggerated thoracic curvature.

Lordosis is an exaggerated lumbar curvature.

Scoliosis is an abnormal medio-lateral curvature of the spine.

Spondylolisthesis is an anterior displacement of one vertebra on another.

Spondylosis is arthritic degeneration of the spine.

A *prolapsed intervertebral disc* (PID) is a condition whereby the disc protrudes posteriorly into the neural canal. This may be due to trauma or arthritic changes. The disc may impinge on nerves causing pain and weakness. The commonest site for PID is the disc between the fourth and fifth lumbar vertebrae and that between the fifth lumbar vertebra and the sacrum.

Fractures and dislocations of the spine. Suspected bony injury to the spine must be treated with extreme caution because of the close proximity of the spinal cord. Common sites of fracture are the twelfth thoracic and first and second lumbar vertebrae in compression-type injuries, e.g. a fall from a height onto the feet. A dislocation of the cervical vertebrae may occur due to acute flexion injuries, e.g. whiplash injury.

SELF–TEST

1 List the functions of the vertebral column.
2 Distinguish between the primary and secondary curves of the spine.
3 Name the two parts of the intervertebral disc.
4 Name the processes of a typical vertebra.
5 Name the structure transmitted in the transverse foramina of a typical cervical vertebrae.
6 Describe the spinous process of a typical cervical vertebra.
7 Name the process of the superior aspect of the body of axis.
8 Describe the shape of the body of a typical thoracic vertebra.
9 Describe the arrangement of the costal facets of a typical thoracic vertebra.
10 Describe the shape of the spinous process of a typical lumbar vertebra.
11 Where is the sacral promontory?
12 What is kyphosis?
13 What is scoliosis?
14 What is spondylolisthesis?

Check your answers against those given at the back of the book.

CHAPTER 7
THE BONES OF THE THORACIC CAGE

THE COSTAL CARTILAGES

The costal cartilages are bars of hyaline cartilage which are attached anteriorly to the ends of the ribs by cartilaginous joints. The first to seventh costal cartilages articulate with the lateral borders of the sternum directly. The eighth, ninth and tenth join together before articulation with the sternum. Those of the eleventh and twelfth ribs are rudimentary.

THE STERNUM (Figs. 40 and 41)

Classification

The sternum is classified as a flat bone.

Situation and articulations

The sternum forms the medial part of the anterior thoracic wall. It articulates with the medial ends of the clavicles and with the costal cartilages.

Bone tissue

The sternum is composed of cancellous bone with a layer of compact bone. The cancellous bone is a rich source of red bone marrow and a sternal puncture may be performed for accurate estimation of the number and status of red blood cells.

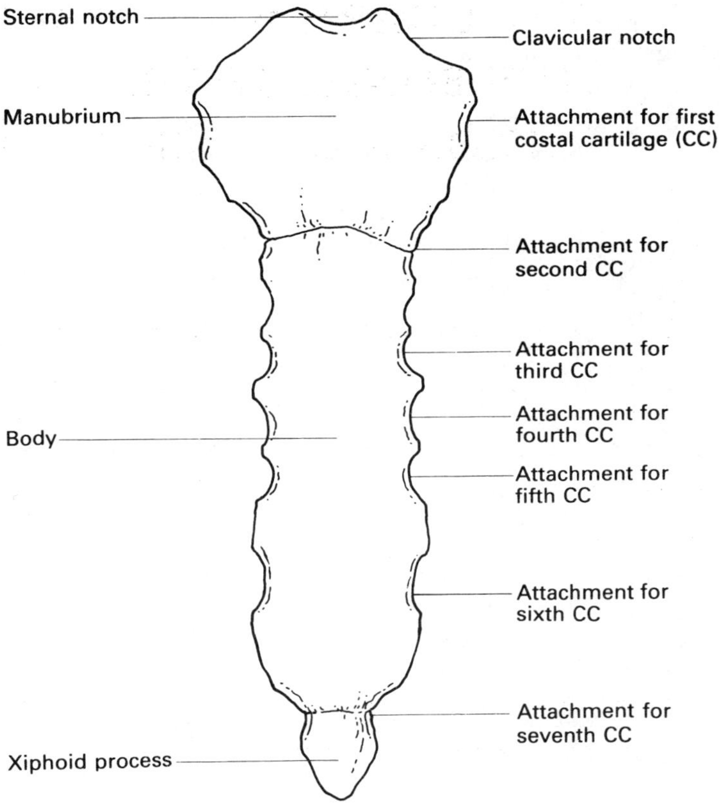

Fig. 40 Sternum — anterior aspect.

Description

The sternum is divided, for descriptive purposes, into three parts: the manubrium, body and xiphoid process.

The manubrium

The manubrium is triangular in shape with the base uppermost. The superior border is marked by a central indentation called the sternal notch. On either side of this is a facet, for articulation with the clavicle, termed the clavicular notch. The lateral borders bear one full notch for attachment of the first costal cartilage and a half notch for attachment of the superior portion of the second costal cartilage. The inferior border articulates with the body of the sternum, forming a prominent transverse ridge called the sternal angle or the angle of Louis.

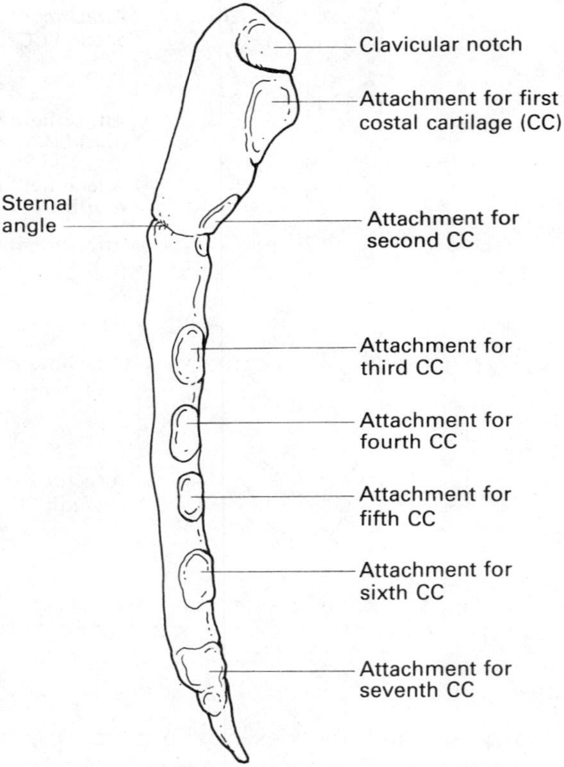

Fig. 41 Sternum — lateral aspect.

The body

The body of the sternum is described as being dagger shaped. It is fused from four segments forming transverse ridges which are usually palpable. It is slightly concave anteriorly from side to side. The lateral border bears a half-facet for attachment of the inferior portion of the second costal cartilage and whole facets for the attachment of the third, fourth, fifth and sixth costal cartilages. Inferior to these facets is a half-facet for the attachment of the superior portion of the seventh costal cartilage. The lower border articulates with the xiphoid process, forming a cartilaginous joint.

The xiphoid process

The xiphoid process is triangular in shape with the base uppermost. It usually ossifies in early adulthood but sometimes remains cartilaginous. It bears a half-facet for attachment of the lower portion of the seventh costal cartilage.

Blood supply

Sternal branches of the internal thoracic (mammary) arteries drain to the internal thoracic (mammary) veins.

Nerve supply

Innervation by branches of the intercostal nerves.

Ossification

The sternum ossifies from a variable number of centres. The manubrium ossifies from one, two or three centres which appear in the fifth month of intrauterine life. The body ossifies from approximately seven centres which appear between the fifth and sixth months of intrauterine life. The xiphoid process may begin to ossify in the third year or much later in life. The centres unite between puberty and the twenty-fifth year, except that the body and manubrium usually remain ununited and the xiphoid process may remain cartilaginous throughout life.

Pathology

Depression of the sternum may occur due to a congenital abnormality or because of trauma. Fractures of the sternum are rare because of the elastic nature of the costal cartilages, but direct trauma may cause a posterior displacement of the sternum. If the depression is severe, compression of the mediastinum may occur.

THE RIBS

Classification

The ribs are classified as flat bones.

Situation and articulations

There are 12 pairs of ribs. They articulate posteriorly with the thoracic vertebrae, curve to form the posterior and lateral bony thorax and are then attached to the costal cartilages anteriorly. The degree of curvature decreases from the first to the twelfth rib. The first to seventh ribs inclusive are called true ribs because they attach to the sternum via individual costal cartilages. The eighth to twelfth ribs inclusive are called false ribs. The costal cartilages of ribs eight, nine and ten join before attachment to the sternum, and the eleventh and twelfth ribs are free. Ribs three to nine are typical ribs and may be described together. Ribs one, two, ten, eleven and twelve are atypical.

Bone tissue

The ribs are cancellous bone with a layer of compact bone.

Description (Fig. 42)

A rib consists of a long, curved shaft with anterior and posterior extremities.

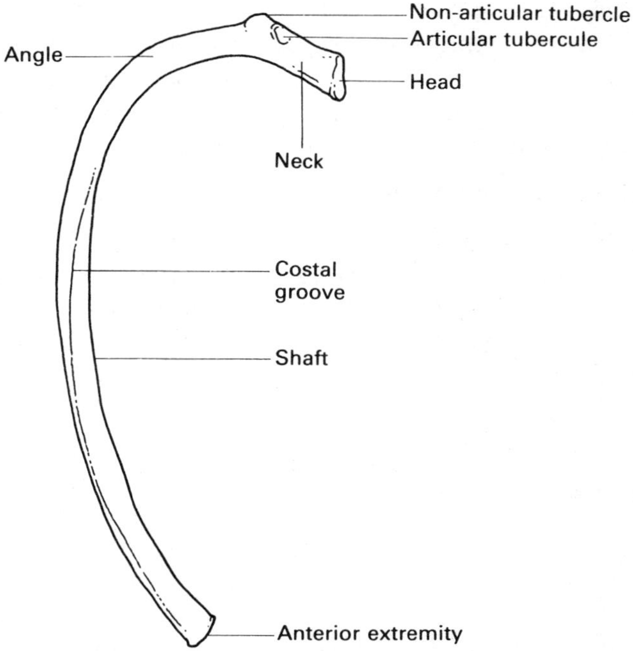

Fig. 42 Typical rib of the left side — inferior aspect.

The anterior extremity

The anterior extremity is concave to receive the appropriate costal cartilage.

The shaft

The shaft forms the greater part of the rib and is situated anterior to the angle. The inner surface is marked by the costal groove, in which lie the intercostal vessels and nerves. The superior and inferior borders of the rib give attachment to the intercostal muscles.

The posterior extremity

The posterior extremity consists of a head, neck and tubercle.

The *head* bears two facets. The lower articulates with the body of the numerically corresponding thoracic vertebra. The upper articulates with the body of the thoracic vertebra above. Between the facets is a crest which is in contact with the intervertebral disc.

The *neck* is a slight constriction separating the head from the tubercle.

The *tubercle* is situated on the external aspect of the rib and is composed of two parts. The articular tubercle forms a joint with the transverse process of the numerically corresponding thoracic vertebra. The non-articular tubercle is roughened for muscle attachment.

Atypical ribs

The *first rib* is short, flat and broad. The head bears a single facet for articulation with the body of the first thoracic vertebra. The superior surface bears the scalene tubercle for insertion of the scalenus anterior muscle. There is no costal groove.

The *second rib* is twice the length of the first but is of similar shape. The outer surface of the midshaft bears a roughened tubercle for attachment of the serratus anterior muscle.

The *tenth rib* has a single articular facet on the head for articulation with the body of the tenth thoracic vertebra.

The *eleventh and twelfth ribs* have a single facet on the head for articulation with the body of the eleventh and twelfth thoracic vertebrae respectively. They do not possess tubercles and therefore do not articulate with the vertebral transverse processes. The anterior ends taper to a point.

Blood supply

Branches from an anastamosis between the anterior intercostal and posterior intercostal arteries drain to the intercostal veins.

Nerve supply

Intercostal nerves.

Ossification

All ribs, except the first, eleventh and twelfth, are ossified from four centres. The primary centre in the shaft appears at the end of the second month of intrauterine life. The three secondary centres, one for the head and one each for the articular and non-articular parts of the tubercle, appear at puberty and unite in the twentieth year. The first rib has three centres: the shaft, head and tubercle. The eleventh and twelfth ribs have two centres: the shaft and head.

Pathology

A cervical rib is a supplementary rib usually arising from the seventh cervical vertebra.

Fractures of the ribs are common in adults. They may have associated complications, e.g. pneumothorax, surgical emphysema, haemothorax.

Flail chest is the name given to a serious condition whereby there are several ribs fractured in more than one place. The flail segment is sucked in during inspiration, thereby causing collapse of the underlying lung tissue.

Rib notchings are indentations of the ribs often due to aortic coarctation. This is because the intercostal arteries become dilated through having to carry a greater volume of blood in an attempt to provide collateral circulation to the aorta, distal to the narrowing.

Ossification of the costal cartilages may occur in old age and occasionally also in young adults. This condition is normally symptomless.

SELF–TEST

1 Name the type of joint formed between the costal cartilages and ribs.
2 State the articulations of the sternum.
3 Name the three parts of the sternum.
4 Where is the sternal angle?
5 Classify the ribs.
6 Differentiate between true and false ribs.
7 Which ribs are atypical?
8 What lies in the costal groove?
9 Name the parts of the tubercle of a typical rib.
10 What is a cervical rib?

Check your answers against those given at the back of the book.

CHAPTER 8
THE SKULL

The emphasis in this chapter is on the skull as a whole and the features visible from various aspects rather than the study of the individual bones of the skull.

The skull is formed by 22 flat and irregular bones articulated together. It consists of the cranium or skull vault and the facial bones. The approximate dividing line between these two portions is the radiographic base-line, an imaginary line between the outer canthus of the eye and the external auditory meatus.

The cranium is formed by one frontal bone, two parietal bones, two temporal bones, one occipital bone, one sphenoid bone and one ethmoid bone.

The facial bones are formed by two zygomatic bones, two nasal bones, two lacrimal bones, two palatine bones, two maxillary bones, one vomer, two inferior conchae and one mandible.

Articulations

The bones of the skull form immoveable fibrous joints called sutures; the exception to this is the temporomandibular joint which is a synovial joint.

There are four principle named sutures:

1 the squamous suture between the parietal and temporal bones;

2 the coronal suture between the frontal and parietal bones;

3 the sagittal suture betwen the right and left parietal bones; and

4 the lambdoid suture between the parietal and occipital bones.

The coronal, sagittal and lambdoid sutures are visible when viewing the skull from above (Fig. 43).

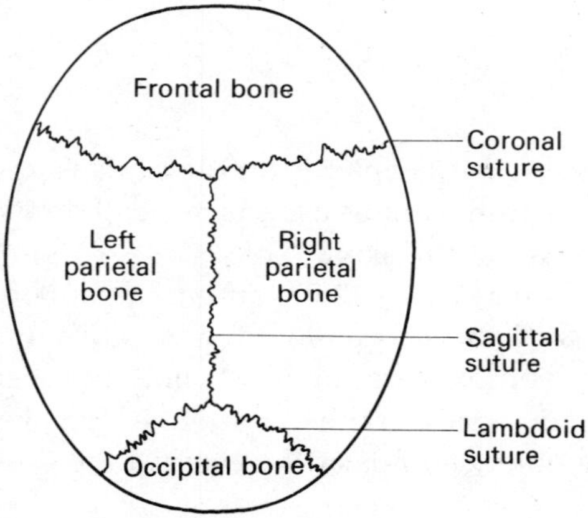

Fig. 43 Skull viewed from above.

At birth, the fusion of the bones is not complete. At the junction of the coronal and sagittal sutures is the bregma which is the site of a membrane-covered gap called the anterior fontanelle. At the junction of the sagittal and lambdoid sutures is the lambda which is the site of a similar, but smaller gap called the posterior fontanelle.

Lateral aspect of the skull (Fig. 44)

Five bones forming the cranium are visible: the frontal, parietal, occipital, temporal and sphenoid.

The visible part of the sphenoid is the greater wing. The visible part of the temporal bone is the squamous part. Extending from the squamous temporal bone is the zygomatic process which unites with the temporal process of the zygoma to form the zygomatic arch. Close to the origin of the zygomatic process is the external auditory meatus. Behind the external

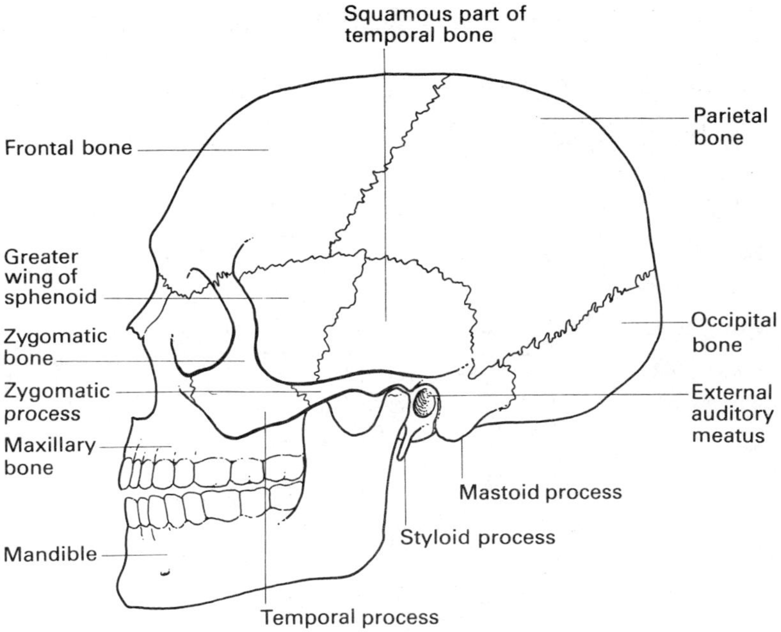

Fig. 44 Left lateral aspect of the skull.

auditory meatus is the mastoid part of the temporal bone which projects downwards, forming the mastoid process. This process contains the mastoid air cells. Anterior to the mastoid process is the styloid process which gives attachment to the stylohyoid ligament.

The facial bones visible from the lateral aspect are the mandible and the zygomatic and maxillary bones.

Anterior aspect of the skull (Fig. 45)

The upper portion of the anterior aspect of the skull is formed by the frontal bone. At the junction of the frontal and nasal bones is the nasion. Superior to the nasion is the glabella, which is situated between the eyebrows. Sweeping laterally from the glabella are the superciliary arches, which are beneath the eyebrows.

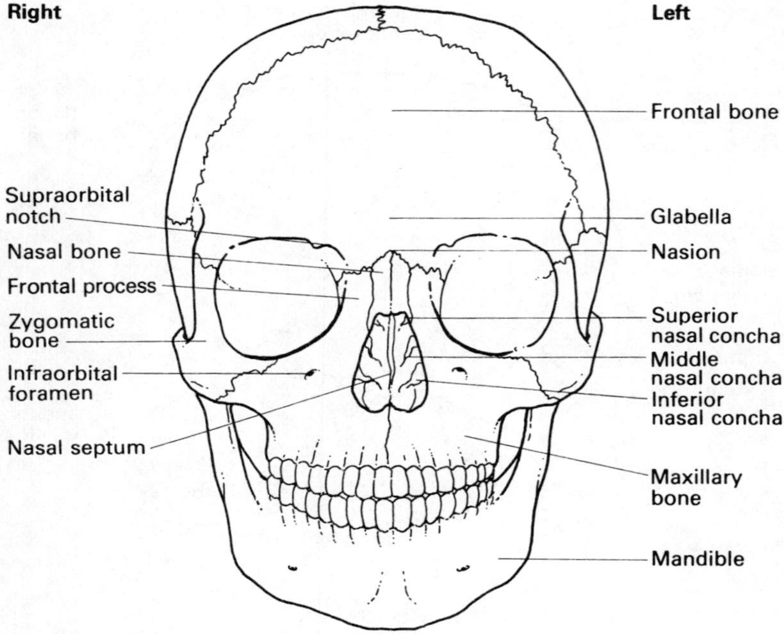

Fig. 45 Anterior aspect of the skull (detail of the orbit omitted).

The upper borders of the orbits, called the supraorbital margins, are marked by the supraorbital notches. The notches are enclosed, forming foramina, which transmit the supraorbital vessels and nerves.

The bony external nose is formed by the nasal bones and frontal processes of maxillae. The nasal cavity is divided approximately in the midline by the nasal septum. Encroaching into the nasal cavity are the conchae: the superior, middle and inferior nasal conchae.

The zygomatic bones are visible inferior and lateral to the orbits.

The maxillary bones form the upper jaw and unite below the nasal cavity. Below the infraorbital margins are the infraorbital foramina which transmit infraorbital vessels and nerves.

The inferior portion of the anterior aspect of the skull is formed by the mandible.

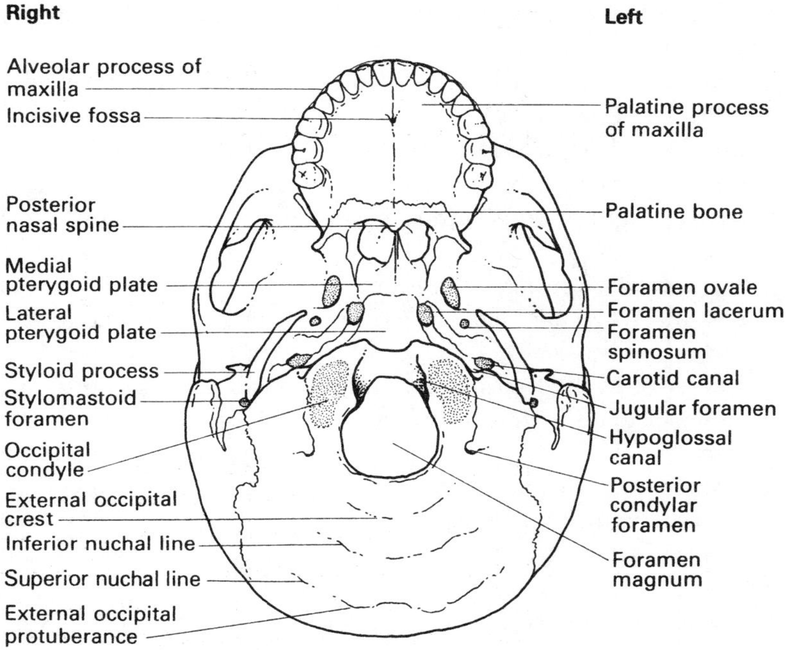

Fig. 46 Inferior aspect of the skull.

Inferior aspect of the skull (Fig. 46)

The anterior part of the inferior aspect of the skull is formed by the hard palate and alveolar processes of the maxillae. The hard palate is formed by the palatine process of maxilla and palatine bones. Its posterior margin bears the posterior nasal spine. Anteriorly, the incisive fossa transmits vessels and nerves. The alveolar process of maxillae is horseshoe shaped and contains the upper teeth.

Posterior to the hard palate is the pterygoid process of the sphenoid bone consisting of medial and lateral plates. Lateral to the pterygoid process on either side is the infratemporal surface, in which are situated two important foramina. The foramen ovale transmits the mandibular division of the trigeminal nerve. The foramen spinosum transmits the middle meningeal artery.

The other foramina in the middle portion of the inferior aspect of the skull are as follows:
Foramen lacerum, which is mostly covered and transmits nothing of significance.
Carotid canal, which transmits the internal carotid artery.
Jugular foramen, which transmits the inferior petrosal sinus, internal jugular vein and glossopharyngeal, vagus and accessory nerves.

Posteriorly is situated the foramen magnum, which transmits the spinal cord and coverings, spinal accessory nerves and vertebral arteries.

Anterior to the foramen magnum are the occipital condyles, which articulate with the superior articulating facets of the first cervical vertebra. Each occipital condyle is pierced anteriorly by the hypoglossal canal (sometimes called the anterior condylar foramen), which transmits the hypoglossal nerve. A posterior condylar foramen may be present and may transmit a small vein.

Lateral to the occipital condyles is the styloid process. Near to the base of this process is the stylomastoid foramen, which transmits the facial nerve and stylomastoid vessels.

Posterior to the foramen magnum is the external occipital crest and external occipital protuberance. The superior and inferior nuchal lines give attachment to muscles and ligaments.

Interior of the base of the skull (Fig. 47)

The interior of the base of the skull is divided into three portions: the anterior, middle and posterior cranial fossae.

The anterior cranial fossa

The anterior cranial fossa contains the frontal lobes of the cerebrum. Medially a sharp projection of the ethmoid bone is visible. This is called the crista galli. On either side of the crista galli is the cribriform plate of ethmoid, which is perforated for the transmission of filaments of the olfactory nerve. Lateral to the cribriform plate is the orbital plate of frontal bone and

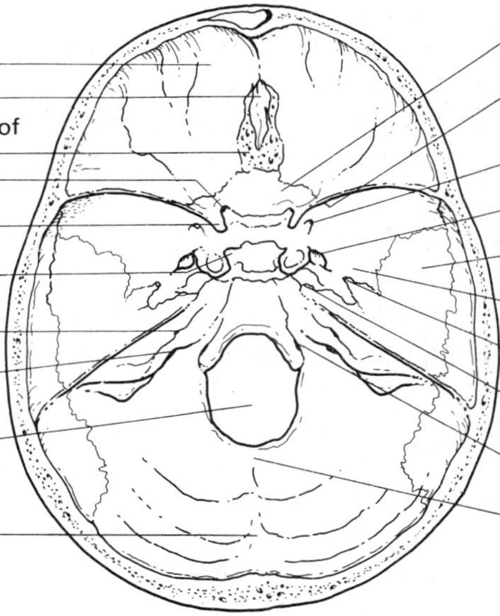

Fig. 47 Interior of the base of the skull.

posterior, the lesser wings of the sphenoid bone can be seen overhanging the middle cranial fossa. Each wing terminates postero-medially in a process called the anterior clinoid process.

The middle cranial fossa

Inferior to the anterior clinoid process on either side is the optic foramen which transmits the optic nerve and ophthalmic artery. Between the optic foramina is the optic groove, in which lies the optic chiasma. The sella turcica or pituitary fossa are the names given to the deep depression which houses the pituitary gland. The posterior wall is formed by the dorsum sellae with projections called the posterior clinoid processes. The pituitary fossa is formed by the body of the sphenoid bone. The lateral part of the middle cranial fossa is formed by the greater wings of sphenoid and temporal bones. The foramina of the middle cranial fossa are as follows.

Superior orbital fissure, which transmits the ophthalmic veins, ophthalmic division of the trigeminal nerve and occulomotor and the trochlear and abducent nerves.
Foramen rotundum, which transmits the maxillary division of the trigeminal nerve.
Foramen ovale, which transmits the mandibular division of the trigeminal nerve.
Foramen spinosum, which transmits the middle meningeal artery.
Foramen lacerum, which does not transmit anything of significance, although the internal carotid artery lies on it.

The posterior cranial fossa

The foramen magnum dominates the posterior cranial fossa. This foramen transmits the spinal cord and coverings, accessory spinal nerves and vertebral arteries. The hypoglossal canals or anterior condylar foramina are visible. They transmit the hypoglossal nerve. Posterior to the foramen magnum is the internal occipital crest and the internal occipital protuberance. Lateral and anterior are two foramina: the jugular foramina. Each foramen transmits the inferior petrosal sinus, internal jugular vein and glossopharyngeal, vagus and accessory nerves. The internal auditory meatus on either side transmits the internal auditory vessels and auditory and facial nerves. The posterior cranial fossa is formed by the temporal and occipital bones.

THE ORBITS (Fig. 48)

The orbits are two quadrilateral, pyramidal concavities situated at the superior and anterior part of the face. Each consists of a base, apex, roof, floor, lateral wall and medial wall. The base forms the orbital margin and the apex is directed posteriorly and medially.

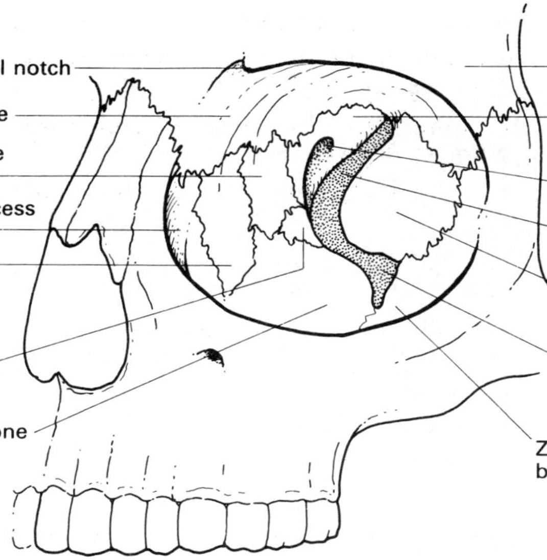

Fig. 48 Antero-lateral aspect of the left orbit.

The base

The orbital margins are formed by frontal, maxillary and zygomatic bones, as illustrated in Fig. 48. The upper orbital margin is marked by the supraorbital notch and is enclosed to form a foramen transmitting supraorbital vessels and nerves.

The roof

The roof is thin and slightly concave. It is formed by the frontal bone and lesser wing of sphenoid. Antero-laterally is the lacrimal fossa in which the lacrimal gland is situated. At the junction of the roof with the medial wall is the optic foramen which transmits the optic nerve and ophthalmic artery.

The medial wall

The thin medial wall is formed by the frontal process of maxilla, lacrimal bone and orbital plate of the ethmoid bone. Anteriorly the medial wall is grooved for the lacrimal sac.

The floor

The floor is triangular in shape and is formed by the orbital process of the palatine bone and maxillary and zygomatic bones. It forms the roof of the maxillary antrum. Posteriorly, at the junction of the floor and lateral wall, is the inferior orbital fissure which transmits the maxillary division of the trigeminal nerve and infraorbital vessels.

The lateral wall

The lateral wall is the thickest part of the orbit. It is formed by the greater wing of sphenoid, zygomatic process of the frontal bone and frontal process of the zygomatic bone. Posteriorly, the lateral wall is separated from the roof by the superior orbital fissure. This fissure transmits the occulomotor, trochlear and abducent nerves, the ophthalmic division of the trigeminal nerve and the ophthalmic veins.

The apex

The apex is formed by the superior orbital fissure.

THE NASAL CAVITIES (Fig. 49)

The nasal cavity is an irregularly shaped cavity situated above the mouth and below the anterior cranial fossa. It is divided into right and left cavities by the nasal septum. This septum usually deviates to one side so that the right and left nasal cavities are of a different size. Each cavity consists of a roof, floor, medial wall and lateral wall.

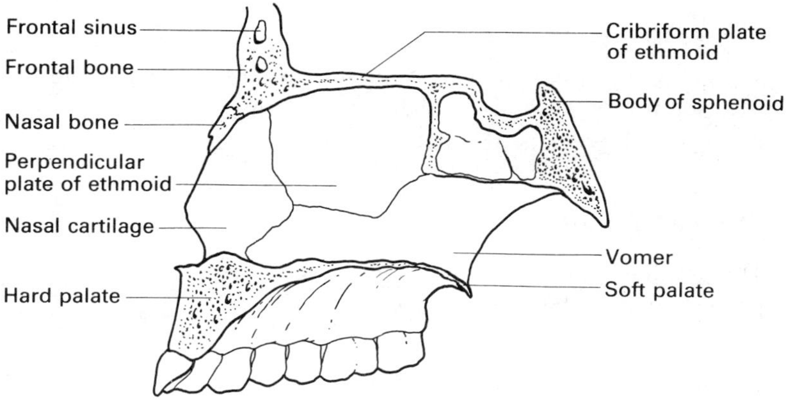

(a)

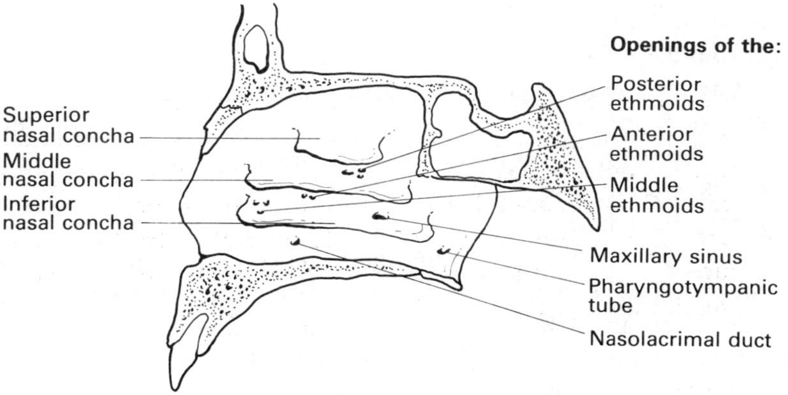

(b)

Fig. 49 (a) Medial aspect of the nasal cavity. (b) Lateral aspect of the nasal cavity to show the conchae and openings.

The roof

The anterior part of the roof is formed by the frontal and nasal bones and also by the nasal cartilages. Medially, it is horizontal and formed by the cribriform plate of the ethmoid bone. Posteriorly, it is formed by the body of the sphenoid bone and is perforated by the opening of the sphenoid sinus.

The floor

The floor is formed by the upper surface of the hard palate, i.e. the palatine process of maxillae and palatine bones. Posteriorly, it is formed by the soft palate.

The medial wall

The medial wall is the nasal septum. It is composed of the perpendicular plate of ethmoid, vomer and cartilaginous nasal septum.

The lateral wall

The lateral wall is irregular and is formed by the medial pterygoid plate of sphenoid bone and parts of the palatine, ethmoid, lacrimal, maxillary and nasal bones. Projecting into the cavity are the nasal conchae: superior, middle and inferior. The superior and middle nasal conchae are projections of the ethmoid bone. The inferior nasal concha is a separate bone. The conchae divide the lateral part of the nasal cavity into four parts. Above the superior nasal concha is the sphenoethmoidal recess. Between the superior and middle nasal conchae is the superior meatus. Between the middle and inferior nasal conchae is the middle meatus. Below the inferior nasal concha is the inferior meatus. Openings into the lateral wall are as follows.

Superior meatus is the site of the openings of the posterior ethmoid sinuses.

Middle meatus is the site of the openings of the anterior ethmoid sinuses, middle ethmoid sinuses, maxillary sinuses and frontal sinuses.

Inferior meatus is the site of the opening of the nasolacrimal duct.

In addition to these, the posterior aspect of the lateral wall bears the opening of the pharyngotympanic tube.

THE ACCESSORY NASAL SINUSES

The accessory nasal sinuses are air-filled cavities within certain bones of the skull. Their function is to add resonance to the voice and to lighten the head. The sinuses are absent at birth and develop over the years before puberty in the frontal, ethmoid, sphenoid and maxillary bones.

The frontal sinuses

The right and left frontal sinuses are situated between the inner and outer tables of the frontal bone. They are divided by a septum which is rarely in the midline and therefore the right and left sinuses are of a different size. Each is approximately triangular in shape with the apex directed towards the nasion. There may be incomplete partitions present which divide each into portions. Each opens into the middle meatus of the nose via the frontonasal duct, although sometimes the duct joins with that of the anterior ethmoid sinuses.

The ethmoidal sinuses

The ethmoidal sinuses lie in the ethmoidal bony labyrinth, between the orbit and nasal cavities. Incomplete bony septa divide them into three groups; anterior, middle and posterior. The anterior and middle groups open into the middle meatus of the nose and the posterior group opens into the superior meatus.

The sphenoid sinuses

The right and left sphenoid sinuses are situated within the body of the sphenoid bone. They are divided by a septum which is rarely in the midline and thus the right and left sinuses are of a different size. Their dimensions are very variable, but it is normal for them to extend back inferior to the sella turcica. They open into the upper posterior part of the lateral nasal cavity — the sphenoethmoidal recess.

The maxillary sinuses

The right and left maxillary sinuses are the largest of the accessory nasal sinuses. They are pyramidal in shape with the apex directed inferiorly. The medial wall of each forms part of the lateral wall of the nasal cavity. The roof of each forms part of the floor of each orbit. Each opens into the middle meatus of the nose.

THE MANDIBLE (Fig. 50)

Classification

The mandible is classified as an irregular bone.

Situation and articulations

The mandible is the bone of the lower jaw and is the only moveable bone of the skull. It articulates with the temporal bone to form the temporomandibular joint.

Bone tissue

The mandible is cancellous bone with a layer of compact.

Description

The mandible consists of a body, two rami and two processes.

The body

The body is horseshoe shaped. It forms in two halves and unites in the midline at two years of age, forming the symphysis mentis. The upper border forms the alveolar margin for the lower teeth. On the external surface near to the symphysis mentis are two roughened areas called the mental protuberance and mental tubercle. Lateral to the symphysis mentis on either side is the mental foramen which transmit vessels and nerves.

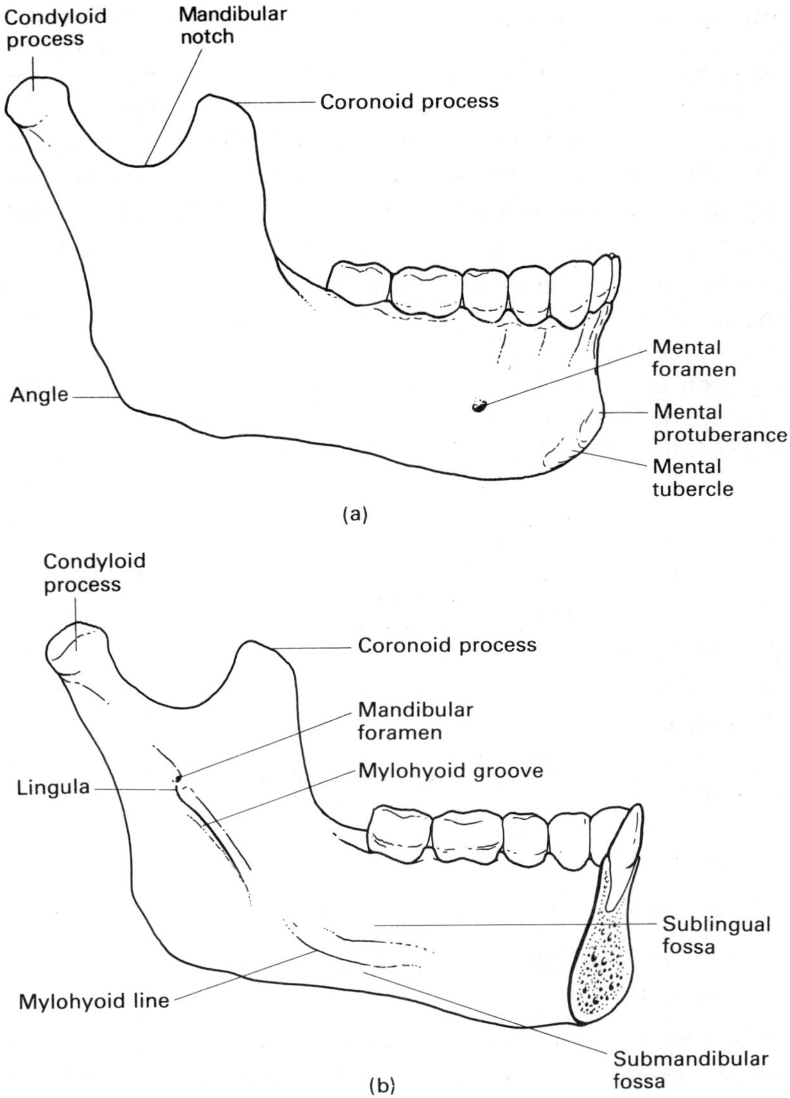

Fig. 50 Mandible — external (a) and internal (b) aspects.

The internal surface is marked by the mylohyoid line. Below this line is the submandibular fossa; above the line is the sublingual fossa.

The rami

The rami are quadrilateral in shape and join the body at the angle of the mandible. The external surface is ridged for attachment of the masseter muscle. The internal surface bears the mandibular foramen. This foramen transmits vessels and nerves into the mandibular canal which opens into the mental foramen. The opening into the mandibular foramen is partially covered by the lingula. Extending from the lingula to the body is the mylohyoid groove.

The processes

The processes are called the coronoid and condyloid processes. The coronoid process is anterior and inferior to the condyloid process. It is directed superiorly and anteriorly and gives attachment to the temporalis muscle. The condyloid process has a head and neck. The head is smooth and oval in shape to articulate with the temporal bone, forming the temporomandibular joint. Between the two processes is the mandibular notch.

Blood supply

A branch of the external carotid artery drains to the external jugular vein.

Nerve supply

The mandibular branch of the trigeminal nerve.

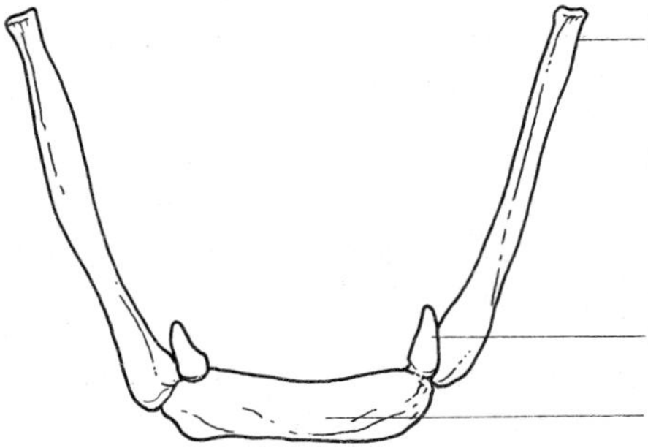

Fig. 51 Anterior aspect of the hyoid bone.

THE HYOID BONE (Fig. 51)

The hyoid bone, situated in the front of the neck, is classified as an irregular bone. It is unique in that it has no bony articulations. It is U shaped, consisting of a body and four processes called horns or cornua: two greater horns and two lesser horns. It gives attachment to 12 muscles, three ligaments and a membrane. It functions as a base for the tongue and aids in mastication, deglutition and phonation.

PATHOLOGY OF THE SKULL

Fractures. Trauma to the skull frequently produces a linear fracture which travels along the line of least resistance. Because the base of the skull is more fragile than the vault, it is often the site of fracture. A direct blow to the head may produce a depressed and/or comminuted fracture.

A *calcified pineal body* is not significant except as a means of diagnosing a space-occupying lesion which may displace the pineal gland.

Raised intracranial pressure is a condition which may produce bony changes in the skull. The venous channels enlarge, as does the foramen spinosum which transmits the middle meningeal artery. The posterior clinoid processes frequently erode and the pituitary fossa may enlarge. If previous to the fusion of the sutures, then widening of the joints will be visible.

Paget's disease is an idiopathic condition. In the early stages the bones become porotic but then they thicken, becoming more dense. The trabecular pattern widens, giving the skull vault a blurred appearance.

Meningioma is a benign tumour of the meninges. It may cause sclerosis of the surrounding bone tissue.

Acoustic neuroma is a tumour of the auditory nerve and may cause an enlargement of the internal auditory meatus.

Acromegaly is a condition due to the oversecretion of growth hormone in an adult. Radiography of the pituitary gland may show an abnormality and the mandible may show an increase in size.

Cholesteatoma is a benign tumour of the middle ear due to overgrowth of the epithelium. It may contain cholesterol.

SELF–TEST

1 What is the name of the type of joint formed between the bones of the skull?
What is the exception to this?
2 Name the bones of the cranium visible from the lateral aspect.
3 Where is the nasion?
4 What does the cribriform plate of the ethmoid bone transmit?
5 Name the bones forming the hard palate.
6 Name the structure(s) transmitted by the foramen spinosum.
7 Name the structure(s) transmitted by the foramen magnum.
8 Name the fissures within the bony orbit.
9 Name the parts of the nasal septum.
10 List the accessory nasal sinuses.
11 Name the processes of the mandible.
12 What is acoustic neuroma?

Check your answers against those given at the back of the book.

ANSWERS TO SELF-TESTS

CHAPTER 1

1 Connective or skeletal connective.
2 Hyaline, fibrous and elastic.
3 Chondrocytes and chondroblasts.
4 Nutrition, repair and appositional growth.
5 Osteoblast, osteocyte and osteoclast.
6 Compact and cancellous.
7 An artery, vein and lymphatic vessel surrounded by areolar tissue.
8 Diaphysis — primary centre of ossification; epiphysis — secondary centre of ossification; and metaphysis — extremity of diaphysis where longitudinal growth occurs.
9 Calcium, phosphorus and vitamins D, C and A.
10 Growth hormone, parathormone, calcitonin, oestrogens, testosterone and thyroxin.
11 Immature bone formed at the stage of callus in the healing of a fracture.
12 Femur — long; vertebrae — irregular; tarsal bones — short; ribs — flat; clavicle — long; patella — sesamoid; and hip bone — flat.

CHAPTER 2

1 Long bone.
2 Head of the humerus with the glenoid cavity of the scapula forming the shoulder-joint; inferior extremity of the humerus with the trochlear surface of the ulna and head of radius forming the elbow-joint.
3 Anatomical neck — constriction separating the head from the tuberosities; surgical neck — constriction separating the upper extremity from the shaft.
4 Tendon of the long head of biceps.
5 Olecranon, radial, coronoid.
6 Shaft is compact surrounding a medullary cavity, extremities are cancellous with a layer of compact bone.
7 Olecranon and coronoid.
8 Lateral border.
9 Radius.
10 Scaphoid and lunate.
11 Long bones.
12 Synovial saddle joint.
13 Trapezium, trapezoid, capitate and hamate.
14 Osteochondritis of the lunate bone.

CHAPTER 3

1 Glenoid cavity with the head of the humerus forming the shoulder-joint; acromion process with the clavicle forming the acromioclavicular joint.
2 Posterior thoracic wall between the levels of the second to seventh ribs.
3 Spine.
4 Pear-shaped, shallow depression.
5 Superior, inferior and lateral.
6 Coracoid process.
7 It is a long bone but does not have a medullary cavity.
8 Sternal end.
9 Acromial end.
10 Clavicular notch of the manubrium of the sternum and the first costal cartilage.

CHAPTER 4

1 Head of the femur with the acetabulum of the hip bone forming the hip-joint; inferiorly with the posterior surface of the patella and tibial condyles forming the knee-joint.
2 Two-thirds of a sphere, smooth except at the fovea.
3 Ligament of the head of the femur.
4 Upper part of the medial condyle.
5 Osteochondritis of the capitular epiphysis of the femur.
6 Quadriceps femoris muscle.
7 Triangular, apex inferior, flattened from front to back.
8 Median ridge.
9 Sesamoid bone which may develop at the back of knee in the gastrocnemius muscle.
10 Lateral condyle.
11 Osteochondritis of the tibial tuberosity.
12 Superiorly with the tibia forming the superior tibiofibular joint; inferiorly with the tibia forming the inferior tibiofibular joint and with the talus forming part of the ankle-joint.
13 Median crest.
14 Second metatarsal.
15 Talus, calcaneum, navicular, medial cuneiform, intermediate cuneiform, lateral cuneiform, and cuboid.
16 Foot deformity whereby the longitudinal arch is lowered, i.e. 'flat feet'.

CHAPTER 5

1 Flat bone.
2 Ilium, ischium and pubis.
3 Superior pubic ramus, inferior pubic ramus, ischial body and ischial ramus.
4 Body of ischium.
5 Protection of the lower abdominal and pelvic organs and weight transference.
6 Promontory of sacrum, pelvic border of ilium and upper border of pubis.
7 Line between the sacral promontory and upper border of the symphysis pubis.
8 Large and round.
9 Congenital dislocation of the hip.
10 Bladder, urethra and rectum.

CHAPTER 6

1 Protection of the spinal cord, support for the head and trunk with flexibility, weight transference, muscle attachment and articulation of the ribs.
2 Primary are present at birth (thoracic and sacrum); secondary develop after birth (cervical and lumbar).
3 Annulus fibrosis and nucleus pulposus.
4 Superior articulating processes (two), inferior articulating processes (two), transverse processes (two), and spinous process (one).
5 Vertebral artery.
6 Flattened supero-inferiorly and bifid.
7 Odontoid process.
8 Heart shaped.
9 Demi-facets on the superior and inferior sides of the body and facets at the free end of the transverse processes.
10 Short, quadrilateral and almost horizontal.
11 Superior and anterior aspect of the sacrum.
12 Exaggerated thoracic curvature.
13 Abnormal mediolateral curvature of the spine.
14 Anterior displacement of one vertebra on another.

CHAPTER 7

1 Cartilaginous joints.
2 Medial ends of the clavicles and costal cartilages.
3 Manubrium, body and xiphoid process.
4 Between the manubrium and body.
5 Flat bones.
6 True ribs are one to seven inclusive (they attach to the sternum via individual costal cartilages); false ribs are eight to twelve inclusive.
7 Ribs one, two, ten, eleven and twelve.
8 Intercostal vessels and nerves.
9 Articular and non-articular.
10 Supplementary rib usually arising from the seventh cervical vertebra.

CHAPTER 8

1 Sutures (immoveable fibrous joints); the exception is the temporomandibular joint, which is a synovial condylar joint.
2 Frontal, parietal, occipital, temporal and sphenoid bones.
3 In the midline at the junction of the frontal and nasal bones.
4 Filaments of the olfactory nerve.
5 Palatine process of maxilla and palatine bones.
6 Middle meningeal artery.
7 Spinal cord and coverings, spinal accessory nerves and vertebral arteries.
8 Superior orbital fissure and inferior orbital fissure.
9 Perpendicular plate of ethmoid, vomer and cartilaginous nasal septum.
10 Frontal, ethmoidal, sphenoid and maxillary.
11 Coronoid and condyloid processes.
12 Tumour of the auditory nerve.

INDEX

Numbers in italics refer to pages on which illustrations occur.